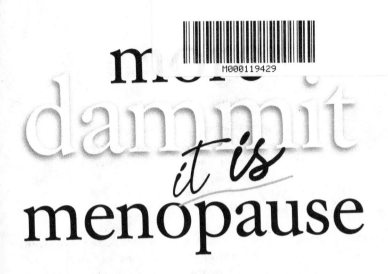

# more dammit *it is* menopause

Meditations for Women to
Achieve Clarity and Confidence
Beyond Their Wildest Dreams

## Sally Bartlett

volume two

**More Dammit … *It IS* Menopause!**
Meditations for Women to Achieve Clarity and
Confidence Beyond Their Wildest Dreams, volume 2
Sally Bartlett
© Copyright 2021
ALL RIGHTS RESERVED

Published by Ginger Books Press
website: SallyBartlett.com
ISBN print: 978-1-7358785-0-8
ISBN eBook: 978-1-7358785-4-6
ISBN audio: 978-1-7358785-5-3

Library of Congress Control Number: 2020921430
Editors: Margaret Ireland; Judith Briles
Book Shepherd: Judith Briles
Cover, interior and eBook design: F + P Graphic Design, FPGD.com

First Edition
Printed in the United States

WOMEN'S HEALTH | MENOPAUSE | MEDITATIONS

To all women

who are at any stage

of menopause.

You are not alone.

Dear Precious—Kathryn,
the world can't wait to
see your unique gifts.
Who are you NOT to share
them with us?

Love, Sally

# AUTHOR'S NOTE

Cordelia's back!

*To protect the privacy of the women whose stories are revealed within my books, I refer to all of them as "Cordelia," after my Great Aunt Cordy (1900-1985). More Dammit ... It Is Menopause! focuses on self-acceptance. Aunt Cordy surrounded me with unconditional acceptance at a young age while going through a challenging period of my life.*

As you can imagine, over the course of 15 years, dramatic changes have taken place in my life. So many that it takes two volumes to tell all the best parts. In Volume One, I share my early awarenesses about peri-menopause and aging in Part One. In Part Two, I share how I came to terms with them and then embraced them like crazy in Part Three. Combined, they became my Varsity Menopause movement.

Isn't that enough? No! It doesn't end there. We never get to coast on the bicycle ride of life. Afterall, the need to adapt and change gears, combined with the willingness to grow continues until we die. What would me, Sally Bartlett, spreading my wings look like? What would my new contributions to my community be?

For this entire volume, I address how the new Sally 2.0 has gone out into the world and spread her wings. I found it had become time. As over 50 advocate Jo Moseley aptly puts it, "It became time for me to spread my own wings and make new contributions to the world."

Moseley's words carried me. Yes, there had been plenty of change-embracing and walking through fears on many levels: physical, intellectual, emotional, and spiritual. Sometimes, I was kicking and screaming in the process. Shifted mindsets, more imperfect food choices, along with mediocre meditation. Then laughter, tears, and love. Each in daily miniscule increments, sometimes one second at a time; sometimes that one second was all I needed. All became my life.

This volume builds on the Varsity Menopause, successful aging foundation, and daily self-care techniques I established and described in Volume One. Then it goes deeper. In essence, Dammit 2 goes deeper. Welcome to Dammit, deeper.

You may wonder … why did I start *More Dammit …* It IS *Menopause!* on 184… and end the first volume on 183? If you read both volumes starting at #1, you will have one entry per day for an entire year. Plus … a BONUS is coming! The companion journal/workbook, due out spring 2021, will include material to last through BOTH volumes.

It's time to ask: What will *your* new contributions to the world be?

You may be well beyond menopause and don't think reading the first volume could possibly be of interest to you. That works fine. But, if you know there are some lingering passions inside, but fear is keeping you from exploring them, reconsider. You are never too old (chronologically or otherwise) to read both volumes—something I highly recommend. If nothing else, at least read the Author's Note so that you know my back story.

My point for you: successful aging requires continual growth and commitment to self-care. That can't happen in isolation. To do this, you need to surround yourself with other Varsity, growth-oriented women to lift you up and remind you how far you've come and that you're well worth the effort.

Walk with me to discover what your new contributions to the world will look like, no matter what your age. You have so much more living to do!

—Sally

### PART IV

# MAKING
# CONTRIBUTIONS
# TO THE WORLD

# 184

## CHANGES IN MY BODY

*My friend Cordelia* (52) called the other day and was lamenting changes in her body which she attributed to menopause. "I looked at my body in the mirror and realized that my body is becoming the body of my mother!" Now, even though these aren't the words I've used to describe the changes in my body that I attribute to menopause, I totally get it.

My 15-year (and counting) journey through peri- and menopause has been just that—a journey. The underlying lesson throughout has been one of acceptance: acceptance of mood swings that make my former PMS mood swings seem amateur; acceptance of night sweats; acceptance of waking up at 3:00 a.m. wired; acceptance of unexpected, ill-timed tears; acceptance of frequently losing my train of thought mid-sentence; and acceptance of how my body changes in less-than-exciting ways, even though I am still choosing the same nutritious food choices and self-loving amounts. For some of these conditions, there are solutions. For some of them, there are not. As for the case of food choices and amounts, the road to acceptance has been a long one.

I had known my clothes fit differently, and I weighed more than I used to for many years. Yes, years. Still, I was unable to drum up the willingness to eat less. The way I saw it, I have been maintaining a 35-lb. weight loss for over 25 years and I'll be damned if I'm going to eat any less than I have always eaten to maintain this weight loss. And that was that. I continued to eat the way I had always eaten. Due to whatever hormone changes had been going on in my body, the amount of food that for years kept me in a body I loved, was now taking me to a body that I didn't love quite as much. Yet I was unwilling to make any changes in my food. I was, however, willing to continue to work toward changing my attitude and loving this new, slightly larger waistline. In other words, contemplating the possibility of embracing the Basketball stomach I feared the most. It has literally taken years of work to accept this.

I don't know what happened, but about a month ago I was eating a meal with friends and family. I was quite engrossed with the conversation and the love I felt for these people, right in that moment. I found myself torn between hearing what everyone had to say and inhaling my meal, to the point where I was frustrated about how to achieve both. Suddenly it occurred to me: "You can take the rest of your food to go!" This may sound overly simple or ridiculous, but it was as if I'd never thought of that. But right then, for whatever reason, something clicked for me. I took the rest of the meal home and have subsequently had the willingness to eat smaller portions ever since. Only 10 years later. My point is, it takes as long as it takes. I usually think in terms of YEARS when I'm thinking of attitude changes.

Dear God,
Please help me to be in acceptance of my body and whatever it is doing today. Also please guide me in choosing nutritious foods in self-loving amounts.

# 185
## LIFE'S TRANSITIONS

*My only child* got his driver's license today. I didn't want to, but a small voice inside suggested I let him drive himself to his martial arts class tonight. As I sat in my bed, unsure of how to feel or act, I decided writing was a better idea than eating. What could I possibly write that would help to assuage these raw, unidentified feelings?

I believe in the power of prayer and meditation and reflection. Whatever one calls it, communication with a power greater than myself has always been healing for me. But talking and listening to a supreme being in my mind has never come easily because my mind is highly active and quite easily distracted. The solution for me has been to write letters to God and have God (aka Big Love) "write" back.

*Dear God,*
*My son got his license today. OMG. I feel like there was*
*a death … like I'm mourning a loss … the loss of being*
*his mom. I still remember driving him home from the*
*hospital after having given birth to him. It was such a*
*huge responsibility—this life. It was so overwhelming that*
*upon arriving home, I promptly directed my husband to*
*get me a large cheeseburger and fries.*

*Now after 16 years of driving him around, he doesn't*
*need me to do that. His dependence on me has decreased*
*a huge amount. I know logically he still needs me a lot,*
*but it doesn't feel like it. It's painful. I feel sad because he's*
*growing up. I miss my baby. He'll never be a baby again.*
*I miss his baby voice, his baby smell, and his baby-sized*
*body. Thy Will Be Done.*
*Love, Sally*

*Dear Sally-Girl,*
*I know, darling. I know you're sad. I know it hurts.*
*I know you miss that baby. You did a wonderful job.*
*And I know you know this, but this is what's supposed to*
*happen. This means you're doing a really good job. But*
*yes, it's still painful. I love you and you can sleep in My*
*arms tonight.*
*Love, God*

# 186

## Trusting My Instincts and Being Patient With the Process

*Today I sent Cordelia* a total of four 3-minute voicemails. As we very often do with each other, I shared my situation. I think I just need a little encouragement from a good and trusted friend. A pep talk would be helpful today.

I patched together my messages, and this is the gist of what I said: "Cordelia, I need to rattle off a whole bunch of thoughts and feelings; otherwise, I cannot move on with my day. My business is coming together, and I have such strong ideas and I know what my next steps need to be and there are a lot of steps that I want to take. I'm finding that between my regular job and my side job, just needing to physically rest, and working out for my sanity, I am falling behind. I am having this avalanche of ideas that I'm writing down. I want to make them happen and put them in place but I'm falling further and further behind. I'm getting frustrated. I need to keep my positivity up. Call me soon. Advice and comforting words would be appreciated."

Dear God,
Please keep directing me on Your will for me and my life course. Help me to continue to believe in myself and to follow my instincts. And give me patience with the process. And Thank You for my friend Cordelia.

# 187

## BEING A GOOD LISTENER FOR MY FRIEND

*For quite some time* my good friend Cordelia (49) has regularly attended aerial class using silk ropes. It makes her heart sing. Yesterday during class, she fell for the first time ever. She called me today wanting to share some things that she has been noticing recently … observations that are bothering her. Here is Cordelia's side of the conversation:

"Lately I have been having a hard time remembering names of aerial tricks we do. Also, if the instructor says the name of a trick, I don't always know what to do. So, there I am up in the air and she must talk me through it, while everyone else in the class knows what to do. I just wonder if, seriously I am starting on early Alzheimer's. Also, there is some strength and ability that I need and I'm feeling stiff in my body, so self-myofascial release is helping. Before each aerial class, I do foam rolling, but it didn't prevent me from a fall in class.

"I didn't really get hurt but I kind of scared myself because we were doing these routines where not only do I have to know the names of things, I've also got to remember these long sequences and some of these other women are already performing. It's exhausting being up there. One move I was able to easily do two weeks ago, but I haven't been able to do it since. More than being scared of actually getting hurt, I think I'm afraid of that old deep-seeded thing of finding out that I can't do this and I'm such a loser and who do I think I am, being 49 years old and trying to do this stuff.

"Never mind that some of these women are my age but have been dancers their entire lives or they're competitive athletes, of course. But with my recent small weight gain, which isn't even that much, I'm feeling insecure. I had negative feelings coming up about just not belonging … like I don't belong here. I'm out of place here. I shouldn't be here. How dare I or who do I think I am? I felt like crying. Sally, I think I just needed to talk to you and tell you about it because I'm not going to let it get me down. I'm just gonna keep fucking going despite that horrible feeling."

Dear God,
What is going on with my friend? Please give me the ability to be strong for Cordelia and for myself as we embrace new chapters in our lives. Help me with my listening skills. I want to be a good listener and encourager to my friends and other women, to support them with Your guidance. Thy Will Be Done (TWBD).

# 188

## CRYING, UNREALISTIC EXPECTATIONS & SELF-COMPARISON

*I've felt like crying a lot lately* ... more than usual. I felt like crying when I arrived at my usual exercise class. I had unrealistic expectations of myself during class and compared myself to the other women in class. I thought I had put self-comparison behind me. The same day, I cried in the middle of Sprouts Farmers Market. What is going on with me?

Just when I think I "have menopause down" (lol) I am reminded it's unrealistic to expect I will ever have aging mastered. When things finally become static, I will be dead. Whether it's unscheduled mystery crying or random ridiculous self-comparison with 20-year-old women, may I embrace each unexpected perspective change with grace.

Reflection:
I love the gentle reminder, "There is a God, and I'm not it."

# 189
## CRYING & BABBLING IS RECOMMENDED

*This is a transcription* of a voicemail message from my friend Cordelia (49), who was en route to work in a sleep-deprived, fear-storm-ridden state:

"Hi. It's Cordelia. I have a serious need to … I need a sounding wall …. No, what do you call that? I need a sounding block. I don't know. I need to talk [laughs]. You know I've been working on stuff and I haven't written my mission statement yet but I'm writing ideas down. I'm going to be typing them up this week. I have a lot going on and I feel like on Saturday I worked hard on my house—not perfect but it's like I don't want to leave my house messy. Okay, I'm completely babbling right now. But I did that and then yesterday I got back into running. Umm … I ran on Friday and then I ran again with my friend yesterday. And Saturday night I was feeling so stiff and in so much pain in my hip … in my shoulder … in my back.

"It's not normal for me and it's been going on for too long. I don't know if it's emotional-based or physical-based or food-based or what, so I decided to do Pilates. I got out the STOTT manual and I went through mat Pilates and you know, and I know that freakin' mat Pilates is just awesome. I made sure I did everything right and it felt so good to be doing it and I was like yeah, I can teach this. At the same time, it made it so clear to me how stiff I am, and I just couldn't even believe my back. I knew my hips were going to be sore and kind of weak, especially with the side-lying leg series that is one of my favorites to do before running, but I was so sore! Not necessarily after, but during … like limited range of motion. And it felt good to do it and at the same time it was this huge eye-opener of OMG … aging … going to be 50 … starting this new business … like I'm totally … OMG, I'm totally gonna CRY.

"Oh, F***. [crying] I'm having like total-imposter syndrome. Here I am having all this pain and I'm supposed to be helping people feel better and I do. And so, I was like okay, just chill out. You must rest. And I did—I rested yesterday, and it was good. Then I woke up in the middle of the night and I'm like freaking out. OMG, I haven't bought my domain name yet! I'm too crazy [laughs]. Losing my mind right now. There's my beep. I'll call you back!"

Dear God,
Please give me the willingness to let myself be me in front of another woman. It heals me and gives the other woman permission to do the same.

# 190

## PARENTS AND LETTING GO

*My father was everything* I could hope for in a dad: hardworking; great provider; loved me like crazy. Best of all, he believed in me beyond a shadow of a doubt. In fact, I was so special to him that he talked about me constantly. My cousins were probably sick of hearing about my latest accomplishment. When he was 92, he experienced a TIA (mini-stroke). Not long after that, he and his companion asked me to help him with paying his bills. I began planning to take on the request. After changing his mind multiple times, it became evident something was amiss. After several subsequent lengthy conversations, I learned he suddenly was convinced it was my secret agenda to take over all his assets and move him into assisted living, neither of which was true. And not only that, he was telling these "facts" to everyone and anyone who would listen.

After repeated attempts to exonerate myself, I realized this man was someone I do not know. The amazing man I called my dad is gone forever. The man who was my biggest fan is never coming back. He's been replaced by this fragile man who is easily psychologically bullied and influenced by an unfamiliar woman who mysteriously came into his life by way of a grief group he joined several years ago when my mom died. This is a woman who has verbally bullied him so severely that within a three-month period, he requested I limit my contact with him to only when his companion is out of town. Meanwhile, he continues to tell relatives about how I'm trying to take all his money and move him out of his home.

My brothers and I conducted extensive research on the situation, from every possible standpoint, legal and otherwise. Taking legal action would have been financially prohibitive and would have brought on what I considered undue stress; not only for my father but for me.

To say the situation has hit me hard doesn't come close to describing its impact on me. It has influenced my health, my job, my self-confidence. It has affected me deeply on emotional, physical, and intellectual levels.

Dear God,

Please watch over this man and his companion. I pray for their health, happiness, and prosperity. Please bring me the self-confidence to believe in my heart what I know is true, no matter what they say about me. Thank You for this opportunity truly to let go of what all others think of me on a much deeper level that I ever thought was necessary.

# 191

## THE POWER OF PRAYER

*Feelings come up about my dad often.* Mostly sadness, but sometimes anger as well. Even though I know logically his mind is not functioning as it once did, it still hurts and doesn't make sense. When I find myself composing what I'd REALLY like to read at his memorial service when he dies, I repeat the prayer for his health, happiness, and prosperity.

Prayer changes me at the cellular level. Angry, vindictive feelings and thoughts hurt me, not the other person. Someone told me it's like taking poison and expecting the other person to die.

Dear God,
I sure didn't see this coming with my dad. This pain is unreal. My heart is broken. Please give me knowledge of Your will for me and the power to carry that out. Thy Will Be Done. Please hold me in Your arms tonight.

# 192
## THE VALUE OF LETTER WRITING

*Feelings come up about my dad and our relationship.* The adult part of me knows that it is pointless to speak to him because his brain is virtually unable to retain anything that I tell him for more than the length of our conversation. But the little girl in me who so adored this man from day one just doesn't get it. That's when the power of writing is immeasurable. Even though the intended recipient will never receive my letter, the writing of it heals me.

Writing helps my brain integrate what that little girl is thinking and feeling with reality. Writing helps my brain be at peace. Writing makes my nervous system settle down. It helps my subconscious mind feel "heard" at a deep level. And this writing "exercise" can help me to identify and express my feelings so that I can move through them and still connect with others in my life who are available to connect with.

*Dear Dad,*

*The fact that you continue to blemish me behind my back hurts even more because you simultaneously continue to send me emails claiming you love me. If you loved me, you would not perpetuate lies behind my back. Please choose one or the other. You have every right to your opinion, but if you are going to believe and spread these vicious lies about me, then out of respect for me, please stop sending the contrary emails. Your current MO feels hypocritical, mean, and is very painful for me.*

Dear God,

I feel incredibly sad. I miss Dad so much. It is especially hard on certain days. I am dreading Father's Day this year. Please help me stay in happy memories like watching *Get Smart* together and laughing. Please hold me tight.

# 193
## DEAR DAD …
## A CATHARTIC EXERCISE

*Here is the letter* I want to email to the man I used to call Dad. I will not be sending this letter, because sending it will open a conversation with someone who is in a compromised mental state and is not capable of reasonable thought. It will expose myself to a lose-lose proposition for both of us and it will magnify my sadness. The best boundary for me is to abstain from communication with him today. Yet it's still painful.

> *Dear Dad,*
> *It is painful for me when you accuse me of having a selfish, deviant agenda for your assets and your welfare. I wish we could return to a simpler time when we are laughing about Oreo cookies in our eyes. It is insulting and devastating to be the receiver of these accusations.*

*It is confusing to me as to where these ideas originated. If you've come to these conclusions on your own, I am incredulous and saddened beyond belief. If they have come from another person, it is incomprehensible to me that you would take the word of someone you have known for a short period of time over the word of your own daughter, who has loved and cherished you since she was born. Why did you and Mom choose me to be your co-trustee?*

*For the past three months, I have spent most of my waking moments trying to figure out how to convince you I'm the same person I always was, who loves you dearly, and who would never do anything to hurt you. I have missed work because of this. I have had daily tension headaches because of this. My own life is on hold as I try to ensure the quality of your life.*

*Yet you continue to accuse me of unthinkable, dishonest intentions, regardless of what I say or do. The bank employee told me last Monday that both you and your companion told him that I am trying to steal all your money.*

*When I learned this, it was a breaking point for me. To respect your wishes and maintain my own health, self-respect, and sanity, I am going to step back.*

31

*Thank you for being the amazing, loving father you have been all my life. I have many happy memories.*

*Thank you for your sense of humor. I will always remember watching* Get Smart *with you.*

*Thank you for being a father who raised me to have extreme integrity in everything I do. Such as having someone's back like you had mine by writing a letter to the Bobby Sox organization when I was 11 because my coach spoke to me so harshly I dropped the ball.*

*Thank you for teaching me to stand up for what I believe in. Thank you for teaching me to speak up for myself. I will always cherish these lessons and these times with you.*

*I wish you the best with your companion and I will ALWAYS love you.*

Call to Action:
Is there someone you could write a letter to? Write it today.

# 194
## GENTLE, GENTLE OR WALL OF SELF-KINDNESS

*My friend Cordelia* was out of the workforce for a while as she raised her children. Now that they are in college, she has had some time to think about what she wants to do with the rest of her life. She's studying to renew her real estate license. She commented to me recently that the studying is going more slowly than she remembers it having gone the first time she prepared for the exam. "I have to read each section aloud or it is virtually impossible to retain anything I am reading!" I am right there with her.

Dear God,
Please help me be patient and gentle with myself in this process. Please enable me to respond to my human-ness with the Wall of Self-Kindness. Saying to myself as many times per day as needed, "Gentle, gentle ... I'm right where I am supposed to be. My timing is perfect."

# 195

## TAKING TEMPERATURES & LIMITING BELIEFS

*I was recently chatting* with my friend Cordelia (56) and made the mistake of taking her temperature. When I am looking inappropriately for validation instead of believing in myself, I call it taking your temperature. I was nervous about planning my first workshop. I wanted to just hand her my script and have her read it to me.

"Sally you are gonna knock this out of the park. I love that you are doing this! Way to go! AWARD!" However, when she was supposed to be reading my script, there were actually crickets on the other end of the line.

After the call ended, I had a knot in my stomach and my head started in with "yeah, her lack of response confirms that holding a workshop is a lame idea. Why don't you just forget it?" Ignoring my head, I went on with my day. The next morning, I realized I'd taken Cordelia's temperature. I haven't done that in a while. How cute am I? Upon further thinking, I realized that Cordelia lived in limiting beliefs. Taking someone's temperature is never a good idea anyway, but taking the temperature of a person who lives in limiting beliefs is the worst. She is imposing her limited beliefs on me. Thankfully, limiting beliefs are not contagious unless I give them that power.

Dear God,

Please help me remember not to take people's temperature. And to have conviction that I'm on Your desired life path for me. And not to give power to people who live in limited beliefs.

# 196

## ADULTING – SOMETIMES QUICKLY, SOMETIMES SLOWLY ... GENTLE, GENTLE

*Several years ago,* my husband and I began the process of setting up a living trust with the help of an attorney. We began. It was uncomfortable. There were aspects of the process I did not understand. I felt as if I was not smart enough. My husband balked at spending that much money. Long story short, the process was never completed.

I am happy to report that two weeks ago, we resumed the process. Fifteen years have gone by since our initial attempt! Sometimes quickly, sometimes slowly. This time I am not intimidated by the fact that I will not know all the answers. However, I am dreading the fact that I will be spending a few hours on this today. There are so many other things that seem more enjoyable. This is one of the parts of being an adult that I hate. But I am doing it anyway because it is the responsible thing to do, and because we do not want our son to experience what I have experienced with my own father.

Reflections:

I am not looking forward to this appointment. Please let me be patient and gentle with myself. I'm so proud of myself for completing this self-care action. It takes as long as it takes. Remember, God will be there with me. All I must do is suit up and show up.

# 197

## Setting Up a Living Trust Award!

*It is done. I have a trust.* I have all my paperwork ready for when I die. Incidentally, this attorney was so good. He explained everything so well and was so patient I hardly even cared when I didn't understand something. And I was not at all embarrassed when I had to ask him to explain something a third—or even a fourth—time!

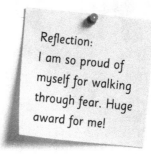

Reflection:
I am so proud of myself for walking through fear. Huge award for me!

# 198

## LIFE ON LIFE'S TERMS, COVID-19 EDITION: PART I

*It's 2020* and here we are in week four of COVID-19 and sheltering in place. Social distancing is the new catch phrase that means no physical contact with anyone who is not in our immediate family. It is suggested that we stay home as much as possible, except for groceries and an outdoor outing one time per day, where we keep a six-foot distance between us and other humans. Many wear gloves and masks. Life as we know it is a little rearranged. There are many adjustments required by all of us. My son is attending the spring quarter of his freshman year of college virtually from home. While he loves college, he is elated to be out of his dungeon of a dorm room.

Anyone who knows me would assume I am over the moon about his return. I am—AND it's a big adjustment for me. I was kind of rocking being an empty-nester. Before

COVID-19, my career was going well. I was doing a lot of new things. I had found my groove. Contrary to what I had expected, I thoroughly enjoyed living alone. My dog and I are amazing roommates.

One thing that my son's return reminds me of is my difficulty staying on task. In between classes, he will often stop by my office to chat. Imagine that. Yet the problem is that once I am interrupted, it takes me a long time to get back to what I was doing. A reminder that my brain doesn't work quite as well as it used to.

On a separate but related note, I feel extremely guilty that I am mentally resisting the idea of dropping everything each time my son wants to chat. I should be so grateful I have a 19-year-old child who wants to talk to me. What kind of mother am I?

*Dear Sally,*
*I love you no matter how fast your brain works. I love you no matter what you are thinking. I love you even though this adjustment is hard for you. I know this makes you want to eat Cheez-Its, and it's okay if you do. But Cheez-Its probably won't improve brain function ... gentle, gentle.*
*Love, Big Love*

# 199

## LIFE ON LIFE'S TERMS, COVID-19 EDITION: PART II

*Although I have no symptoms,* I wonder almost daily if I have the virus, but am in denial. After all, they say some carriers are asymptomatic. I am extremely tired all the time lately. I must let this go. This level of upheaval and life rearrangement we all are experiencing would tire anyone out, irrespective of age. I have lost all sources of income. I am attempting to pivot my clients to virtual sessions, and there is a massive learning curve for all that.

Yesterday I almost lost it in the grocery store. There I was, all proud of myself that I was up and at the grocery store by 6:30 a.m. As I parked the car, it began to rain. I prepared myself with gloves, mask, and glasses. I made a dash from the car to the store. On the way, with the combination of the rain and the mask, my glasses fogged up. I could not see with my glasses on. And I cannot read anything with my glasses off. I was stymied. We have been advised never to touch our face so I couldn't remove my glasses to touch my face. But I had to get to that toilet paper shelf!

You know I got that TP. The whole excursion took twice as long, due to the vision issue. I was very frustrated. I felt old. I kept revisiting the whole experience in my head for a few hours.

*Dear Big Love,*
*Help me to let go of my love of revisiting unpleasant*
*experiences. Yes, that was unpleasant today. But it is in*
*the past. Help me create a new neural pathway in my*
*brain.*

# 200

## Life on Life's Terms, COVID-19 Edition: part III

*My friend Cordelia* (50) left me a voice text today. Like all of us, she is sorting through her personal journey. We check in on each other's roller-coaster of thoughts and emotions almost daily. Today she described her reality as follows:

"I am feeling these very heavy emotions. I know what they are. They are growing pains. I am changing. I am afraid. I am not sure who I will become. Will I like her? I hope she is as awesome as I am now because I like her very much (finally). I know she will be even more awesome. After years of having worked multiple jobs at once, I have been craving downtime like crazy. Now I have it, yet it scares me. Who am I without multiple jobs? Who am I with the social component removed? I know this is good, but it is unfamiliar … uncomfortable. It is a time to focus inward. I will be awesome."

After listening to Cordelia's voice text, I reached her by phone and said, "I know you will be awesome because you already are. Now you will be awesome-squared. I am dying of suspense for the launch of Cordelia 2.0!"

I am honored to hold a space for Cordelia's thoughts and feelings. And I am grateful for her reciprocation in kind.

I can't help but notice the parallels between women's menopausal journeys and their COVID-19 journey. Hmm. I'm thankful for this growth experience times two.

Reflection:
Think about the launch of YOU 2.0. You will be awesome-squared!

# 201

## SECRET FANTASY, UNREALISTIC EXPECTATIONS

*I had the opportunity* to meet by phone with a friend of a friend who is an author and has published many books. I was giddy with excitement, a little nervous as well. She spoke with me for about 30 minutes. She gave me a list of things to do. She gave me constructive feedback on how I could improve on my book, suggesting it needed to be longer, meaning I had to write MORE. She apologized for the blunt manner of her suggestions, to which I quickly responded, "Oh no, not at all. I so value your input." Yet inwardly, I was a little crushed, because my unrealistic expectation of the conversation was as follows: "I love the idea of your book. It's perfect exactly the way it is right now and in fact, I'd like to publish it through my publishing company as soon as possible. Let's get to work. Will an advance help you?"

The call ended and I felt deflated. As is often the case, my expectation of how a situation "should" go is quite different from reality. I immediately wanted to eat something. I wanted to quit working on the book … again. I could not possibly write 60 more pages for my book. No! My answer is NO because I just don't want to.

Instead, I voice-texted my friend Cordelia to express my colossal disappointment. Talking out loud into my phone, I was able to identify my black-and-white, perfectionistic thinking. I decided to pause instead of eating. I decided not to make any decisions about the future of my book right then.

Dear God,
Give me the ability to pause right now and give my feelings and this situation to You. Give me the ability to sit through these uncomfortable feelings instead of quitting like I've done so many times before. Help me to believe in myself and remember that these feelings are just that—feelings. Feelings are not facts.

# 202

## Unrealistic Expectations, the Sequel

*Today I awoke in a completely different mindset* about yesterday's talk with the published author. Funny, yesterday I thought the only thing she said was *your book isn't good enough and it needs more work*. Today, I remember that she also gave me some great suggestions. And because I was willing to pause yesterday, I realized that if she had thought my book was a stupid idea, she never would've given me that constructive feedback. Meanwhile, my friend Cordelia voice-texted me back, saying she related very much. She said that from now on whenever someone gives her constructive feedback, she's going to mentally translate that info to: "I just got told I'm doing a great job." We both made a vow to do that.

Today, I am willing to write 60 more pages for my book. Today that does not sound impossible or unreasonable or unrealistic. Yesterday it was all of that. What a difference a day makes.

*Dear Big Love,*

*Help me to remember to pause when agitated today and ask You for guidance that may come through an unexpected source, such as my friend Cordelia.*

# 203
## GETTING OUT OF MY HEAD

*Every day I walk my dog* for about 30 minutes. Today was no exception. However, just as I was finished with my lap around the park, a train horn sounded in the distance. It even got my dog's attention. Something about the sound of a train moves me. It causes me to stop and take notice. We both stood still and listened to that glorious sound. Once it stopped, I realized I had been completely in my head throughout the entire walk. Suddenly, I noticed the birds. Their songs were equally moving. I stood a little taller. I felt my feet in my shoes. I felt my shoes on the ground. I breathed the air in with renewed awareness. I felt the early morning chill on my face. It was magnificent. Thank you, Nature.

> *Dear Nature,*
> *Help me remember to take time each day to stop and experience life through my five senses. ... to get out of my head and into my feet and my body.*

# 204

## Fit Spiritual Condition

*As I've mentioned,* I've been maintaining a 35-lb. weight loss for over 30 years without dieting. That weight loss and maintenance of it did not just magically happen. It required a daily recommitment to staying current with my feelings, daily being conscious of my thoughts and actions, and a daily willingness to be open to "the new and uncomfortable," whatever they look like. In short, if I am willing to stay spiritually fit, my bouts of unbridled eating are farther and farther apart, and I stay the size I have been for all these years.

*Dear Big Love,*
*Thank You for another day of willingness.*

# 205
## REVISITING DAIRY

*I started hearing things* about dairy and inflammation. I have been fortunate in that I have enjoyed consuming dairy products in moderation all my life.

As I write this entry, I am 60 years into my magnificent life journey. I'd been hearing that dairy can cause inflammation in the aging body for several years, but I didn't want to listen because let's just say, "I love me some dairy." Cheese? Are you kidding me? Sometimes I think about taking a bath in a fondue pot. With all the work I've done on myself for all these years, now you're gonna say dairy and I are breaking up?

About two years ago, I chose not to have dairy for one day, just to prove "they" were wrong about it causing inflammation in the aging body. Guess what? I could feel the difference; I liked the feeling. Consequently, most days, I choose not to have dairy because I like the way I feel. But somedays, because I suffer from ISM (Incredibly Short Memory) and CRS (Can't Remember S***), I decide to eat dairy. Yesterday I ate some delicious organic yogurt as a treat after dinner. Almost as soon as I put the spoon down and licked around the top of the container, I felt this unpleasant mucous-y feeling every time I swallowed. During the night, my hands ached. Today my nose is running and I am not sick. How cute am I? I had to try dairy again just in case something had changed. Today I will choose not to have dairy and I will love the way I feel.

> *Dear Sally-Girl,*
> *It is not the end of the world that you ate dairy.*
> *Remember, I love you not only despite your*
> *imperfections, I love you BECAUSE of them.*
> *Love, God*

# 206

## SOMETIMES MY MIND IS A DANGEROUS NEIGHBORHOOD

*Today as I was picking up my dog's poop,* I noticed it was smaller than usual. Have I mentioned I'm a little bit detail-oriented/anal-retentive/obsessive-compulsive? Before the bag was even knotted and thrown away, in my mind I was already in a veterinary ER situation with my dog having emergency surgery to remove the excessive rope toy strings that were obstructing his digestive tract. Oh, and I'm freaking out about how I was gonna pay that huge bill. LOL. How cute am I?

Call to Action:
If everything was just the way it was meant to be today, think about what you would be free to feel.

# 207

## There Is Always Time to Go to the Bathroom

*I know it sounds crazy,* but sometimes I need this reminder. My memory has gotten so bad that at times I do not want to stop what I am doing because:

I may not remember what I was doing.

I may lose the burst of energy I was experiencing and not be able to get it up again.

*Dear Universe,*

*Please help me to let go of what I accomplish today. Help me to trust that whatever I need to remember will come to me in the right time/ space sequence. The timing of the Universe is perfect.*

Call to Action:
Give yourself permission to stop; permission to rest; and permission to breathe.

# 208

## ACCOUNTABILITY & CLOSING THE KITCHEN

*As a person* with an addictive personality, dinner is the hardest meal of the day for me. Because once that meal is over, there will be no "padding" between my feelings and me. Sometimes I feel like I might die from feelings during that period where I am not eating. Sometimes after having eaten my intended dinner, I get a "better" idea about my original choices. A significant mental debate ensues about whether I have eaten enough for the day or if I need to eat just one more thing ... and what could it be?

This is when I use the tool of closing the kitchen. When this debate drags on, I text a declaration to knowing sisters that my kitchen is closed. They inevitably text back a thumbs-up or a heart. Ninety percent of the time, they will declare their kitchen is closed as well. This strengthens my commitment and reminds me I am not alone, and we are stronger together. Once I proclaim that my kitchen is closed, it is with the understanding that I am brushing my teeth and nothing else will go in my mouth until breakfast. It also means that if I decide to reopen my kitchen, I will text those same sisters back to be accountable.

This accountability tool is invaluable. I cannot tell you how many times taking this small action has relieved me of the urge to eat spontaneously and/or beyond the point of fullness. It reminds me that I strive to eat to live, rather than live to eat. It is indescribably comforting to know that at that very moment, someone else out there feels like I do. I am not a crazy whack job, I am a feelings-based woman who might want to identify her feelings right now, instead of eating over them.

And likewise, when someone else texts me about her closed kitchen, nine times out of ten, I was right in the middle of the same debate myself and this connection gives me the clarity to pause and join the club.

Dear God,
I feel afraid that if I honor my hunger right now, I will feel uncomfortable feelings. Please give me the strength to sit down and write You a letter about my fears, even if it's only one sentence. There's always the option to write more.

On tough days, I have even felt the need to close the breakfast and/or lunch kitchen. Works just as well!

Call to Action:
Ask a safe woman who struggles with emotional eating if she would be willing to be your kitchen-closing accountability partner.
Write a "Dear God, I feel [blank] because [XYZ]" letter.

# 209
## Puppies and HRT

*When I walk my male dog,* people often mistake him for a her. He has unusually large nipples that resemble the nipples of a female dog who is still nursing her babies. When the person commenting seems a little creepy and a little too excited about saying the word "nipples" repeatedly (usually men over 50), I confirm he is male and politely move on. When the person asking feels safe, I will tell the real story (or maybe not).

The truth is, at the time when my dog was a puppy, I was using bioidentical hormone cream prescribed by my OB/Gyn based on lab work that determined my most current hormone levels. The hormone deficits were calculated by the doctor and the prescription was then prepared by a compound pharmacist. Somehow, I missed the part where they told me to use gloves when I applied it to my thighs and then allow it to dry for a while before touching any living being, and to thoroughly wash hands upon glove removal. I had been applying the cream to my forearms with bare hands, and immediately returning to whatever (puppy tending & loving) once I applied the cream in the evening.

From the age of 12 weeks to adulthood, my beloved Wilson had been exposed to my personal blend of HRT. After all, what dog lover can resist rubbing a puppy's belly? My female vet set me straight. Even though gloves, thigh application, handwashing and air-drying became a part of my daily routine from then on, Wilson's nipples remain enlarged to this day.

*Dear Sally-Girl,*
*How were you supposed to know? You did the best you could with the information you had at the time. And by the way, great job having boundaries with whack jobs who make inappropriate comments.*

Dear God,
I feel terrible about unknowingly transferring my hormonal cream to my dog that caused his nipples to enlarge ... and stay that way!

# 2IO

## WHAT I WEIGH IS A MATERIAL THING

Over 35 years ago, a wise woman told me, "What you weigh is a material thing. To lose weight and keep it off, you have to put spiritual growth first." To this day, I still frequently say this to myself. For as long as material gain is at the top of my list of priorities, I have never been able to achieve anything. Nor have I been content. Material aspirations render me incapable of being in the present. The inability to be in the present steals my capacity for spiritual growth.

Call to Action: Remember, life is best lived in the present. Like any new skill, learning to live in the present takes practice and repetition. Every time you find yourself preoccupied with material gain, such as what you weigh or what your body looks like, return to the question, "If everything was unfolding just the way it was meant to today, what would I be free to feel?" This will bring you back to the present. Practice makes progress.

# 2II

## NO ONE EVER TOLD ME RELATIONSHIPS ARE MESSY

*In my grade school years,* I had a hard time making friends. It was my experience that girls were mean and cliquish, and I quickly lost interest in trying to be a "part of." Girl drama often leads to disappointment, hurt feelings, and tears. It seemed like a waste of time. At that time, there was no one in my life to guide me on this. No one to tell me that feelings are healthy, normal, and appropriate ... and inevitable. There was no one to teach me skills to process feelings appropriately. And I had a lot of feelings with no outlet. I began to feel as if something was wrong with me because of all the things I thought and felt. The things I thought and felt never seemed to match the things the kids around me were vocalizing. I mostly kept my thoughts and feelings to myself.

My parents were devoted, loving parents who looked good on the outside and wanted the best for their children.

They did the best they knew how, but no one had ever taught them that feelings are healthy, normal, and appropriate. Feelings are meant to be felt. Feelings pass. How could they have taught me something they had never been taught themselves?

Looking back, this was when I began doing anything I could to avoid uncomfortable feelings. Around 10 years old, I decided it was just too uncomfortable to deal with relationships. Unless someone did everything the way I dictated, I wasn't interested (red flag much?). My social development became arrested from that point on, to some degree.

Being athletic, I was able to "bypass" feelings somewhat by participating in sports. This was much more fun, the release of endorphins felt fantastic, and there was much less drama. I channeled a lot of my energy into sports. I enjoyed being a tomboy for as long as I possibly could.

By the time I got to high school, I wasn't really into being a tomboy anymore, but I still couldn't relate to the way girls treated each other. I remained active in sports but other than that, I was somewhat of a loner by choice. My resistance to participating in the social interaction that would have been appropriate for my age brought on bigger problems. It led to perfectionism, body dysmorphia, and disordered eating.

Dear God,

Help me remember I am always a work in progress. It is never too late to learn relationship skills. I am never too old to improve my communication skills. I am never too old to learn how to appropriately process feelings.

# 212

## ON JUST BEING YOURSELF ...
## MIXED MESSAGES

*There were a few techniques I adopted* as a child to avoid feelings. One technique that worked for years was people-pleasing adults. I usually didn't feel like I fit in with my peers, and preferred interaction with my teachers. I was a teacher's pet whenever possible. During recess, I would stand and chat with the teacher on duty. This worked a lot of the time, except in cases where the teacher was not into me, like Miss May in third grade. She was not at all into my people-pleasing. One day she asked the class their opinion of something. I raised my hand and gave my opinion that was apparently contrary to majority opinion. Miss May disappointedly declared, "Thanks to 'Queen Sally,' the entire class loses recess today!" From that day on, I have been reluctant to give my opinion when asked for fear of possible repercussion.

Dear God,
Please take away my people-pleasing tendencies and give me the courage to be the real Sally.

# 213

## SOCIAL MEDIA ...
## ARE YOU IN THERE, GOD?

*While I enjoy social media* and am quick to see its benefits, it can be problematic for the addictive personality in me. If I did not exercise discipline, I could easily check social media 20 times per day. The problem arises when: I expect to receive validation from it; when I expect to receive approval from it; and when I expect to receive love from it. Ideally, I feel best when my sense of self-value comes

Dear God,
Help me to remember to check my spiritual condition before I check my social media.

from within or from a power greater than myself.

Each time I reach for that phone, I check myself. What do I hope to gain? Connection with my fellow humans? A smile and laughter? A chance to do service for someone else? If I answer *yes* to these questions, then I open the app.

However, if I am asking myself, "Am I loveable? Does anyone love me? Am I doing a good enough job today? Is God in that app?" the app is not going to help me in that moment.

# 214

## MAKE FIVE MISTAKES A DAY
## AND CELEBRATE: PART I

*One of the ways I recover* daily from the crippling disease of perfectionism is not only to allow myself to make mistakes, but to celebrate when I make mistakes. In recent weeks, I have endeavored to pivot my in-person health coaching business to an online health coaching business. There was a time in my life when I would never even attempt such a change because (A) I hate change, and (B) I wasn't an expert on XYZ. Nowadays, I do things anyway.

On my first Zoom session:

- I inadvertently failed to virtually "admit" someone from the waiting room, and she missed the entire class.

- I told the group I would record the session and send it to them, but only recorded my conversation with my business partner instead of the class.

- I forgot half of the planned exercises because I was so nervous.

By the standards I set for myself these days, in just this 50-minute period I was well on my way to meeting my criteria for daily celebration. When my mistakes became evident to me, I smiled and got out the freakin' figurative confetti! Nice job, Sally!

Dear God,
Help me remember that in being human before others, I give them permission to be human as well. What a gift for all of us.

# 21§

## RE-INHABITED NEST SYNDROME:

### PART I

*My son went off to his freshman year of college.* It was hard. I knew it would be. I prepared ahead of time. During the summer leading up to his departure, I learned new skills and prepared to expand my business. I took his imminent departure as a sign that it was time for me to step into a new role. Prior to that, "Sally the Mom" had been the best job I'd ever had in my life. I never wanted that job to end. But I knew it was time. I studied. I stretched out of my comfort zone. I grew. I learned. I grieved.

The dreaded day came when I drove him to college and came home alone. I hadn't been wrong. It was extremely hard; I felt sad. After so many years of thinking as a parent, it was a large adjustment to think as Sally. To schedule my time around what Sally wanted.

But I got through it. It took weeks to get used to the quiet. I let the tears flow. I embraced the whole thing. I shared with other mothers who were in the same place. We cried and laughed together. I did it. I survived. I thrived. I bloomed. I was deliriously happy, discovering what felt like my true self coming out in a way I had previously only imagined. I awoke excited most mornings, with a flurry of creative ideas about how to spend my time and energy.

Just before spring break, COVID-19 happened. My son is doing college on Zoom from home now. So much for the empty nest ….

Dear God,
Thank You for my willingness to be courageous and walk through the unknown. Please give me a fresh dose of willingness to be radically flexible and bend with the unexpected.

# 216

## Re-Inhabited Nest Syndrome, Economizing on Feelings, Fear of Having to Re-Grieve Empty Nest:
### Part II

*I found myself annoyed with him.* Why? We're talking about one of the most good-natured people I know. Anyone who knows me knows how much I adore my son. Something was not right about my attitude. I wrote about it. I talked about it with someone I trusted. It made no sense; still, I couldn't deny my feelings. I wrote and talked some more.

Through this inward-looking journey, I eventually understood my response to this situation better. My friend Cordelia asked me if I was trying to economize on feelings. This is an expression I use when I am trying to avoid feeling my feelings. Nailed it! I don't know why, but even though I have been embracing all my feelings (eventually) for over 30 years, I still wish I could avoid feelings. I am aware that doesn't make sense, but it's the truth. It's related to that small remnant of perfectionism that hasn't gone away. Deep down, part of me wishes I didn't have to be in relationships because they involve feelings. Cordelia reminded me that relationships are kind of the whole point of life. Oh, yeah.

Having said that, on some level I am blemishing my son by criticizing him or judging him harshly. Sometimes I blemish a person in an effort not to connect with him or her. I know how painful it will be when he leaves again, so my immature self thinks that if I don't connect with him, I can avoid feeling all that pain again. I don't want to do Empty Nest 2.0.

I sat down with my son to talk. I described where I was coming from without apologizing. Because I have raised a kid with communication tools, it was a good conversation. He reminded me that we are both still figuring out what this will look like. The communication channel remains open and this chapter continues to unfold. What a miracle.

Call to Action:
Take a nonjudgmental look within. Is there any economizing of feelings going on in your head? Talk about them with your health-care provider or a safe friend.

*Dear Big Love,*

*Remind me that it is impossible to economize on feelings (but nice try!). Remind me that I will be able to handle whatever feelings come my way in my current situation. I have You and I have amazing friends who hold a place for my precious feelings.*

# 217

## RE-INHABITED NEST SYNDROME, FUTURE TRIPPING: PART III

*I remember vividly* how painful it was when my son went off for college the first time. Now that shelter-in-place has brought him home for a while, I am future-tripping that his imminent departure again will be just as painful for me. While some people are joyful for some extra serendipitous time with their child, I just naturally future-trip.

Thankfully, I have people in my life who can reel me back in by gently reminding me it behooves me to stay in the present.

> *Dear Big Love,*
> *How cute am I the way I love to future-trip. Please bring me back and give me the ability to bloom where I am planted. And thank You for never tiring of gently bringing me back to the now. The point of power is in the present moment.*

Call to Action:

Check in with yourself for 60 seconds. Notice your feet. How they feel in your shoes or on the surface upon which you are standing. Feel your hips above your ankles, your shoulders over your hips, your ears over your shoulders. Where are you right now? Have you been doing any future-tripping lately? Breathe.

# 218

## Don't Interrupt What I'm Doing ... It Will Take Me 60-120 Minutes to Get Back to What I Was Doing

*Three things that have challenged me* since my early 40s are memory, train of thought, and mental momentum. When I first experienced forgetting things (such as purse and keys) and losing my train of thought, I would become extremely frustrated and upset about it. I experienced negative self-talk about my lack of efficiency. My recovery from perfectionism relapsed a bit. It took some time to embrace these issues and remember that I am still lovable, even though I am imperfect.

Observing older friends' behavior around this, I eventually softened. Now I can even laugh when I lose my train of thought. I pause and smile, trusting the thought will return at just the time it is meant to. I have even devised little memory tricks. If I want to remember to take something with me when I leave, I will hang it on the doorknob of the door that leads to my car.

My biggest challenge, however, is what I call mental momentum. It takes me quite some time to start when I sit down to a task. I am easily distracted by laundry-folding, social media, checking my emails, clicking links, and before I know it, an hour has gone by. This, coupled with the fact that everything takes me longer than it once did, makes me way less efficient than I once was. I dread taking a break for lunch at noon because it may be 3:00 p.m. before I resume a desired task. Or I may never get back to that task at all!

Along those same lines, if my son comes over (to my room) from college (down-the-hall-shelter-in-place learning) to tell me about the exam he just took, that harmless interruption of my mental momentum takes a heavy toll on me. It could be 30 minutes before I am back on track.

*Dear Big Love,*
*Thank You in advance for helping me wear my day like a loose garment; for helping me get back on track after interruptions; for enabling me to let go of my timing. And thank You for never tiring of gently bringing me back to the now. The point in life is the relationships with the people; not the amount I produce.*

Call to Action:
Be willing to turn over one of your expectations for yourself today to a positive Universal Power. Now you can let that expectation go for another day. Breathe.

# 219
## BOUNDARIES

*Of course,* I know that I can always improve on being flexible. And the same goes for open-mindedness. And I am constantly reminded of my tendency to be critical and judgmental. But underlying all of these is my need to discern the necessary balance among these traits and having boundaries.

The case of my reinhabited nest syndrome situation is an example of this. It has been helpful to look within and determine how best to divide my time between "me" time and "we" time with my son. He is not the same teenager he was when he left for college and he doesn't want to be treated as such. Each morning, we discuss a loose framework for what each of our days looks like. I've realized that when I don't want to be interrupted, I can close my door. I know that sounds obvious to some, but sometimes I have a slow processing speed.

*Dear Big Love,*

*Please keep reminding me that each new situation I encounter needs to be evaluated. What boundaries do I need to set for myself? Please guide me on the delicate balance in me between a doormat and a bulldozer.*

# 220

## INTIMACY & A FAULTY PICKER

*I am intense.* I think a lot about things. I constantly seek inner growth. That's how I am wired. I crave intimate relationships. By "intimate," I don't necessarily mean sex, although I'm not opposed to that. I mean me-being-me-and-letting-you-see-me. Not everyone seeks or even desires relationships with the same level of intimacy that I seek. I have spent a lot of life picking people to be in relationships with who either do not want or are incapable of being in a relationship at the level I want. It has been an ongoing life lesson for me to honor people where they are and honor me where I am. Another huge life lesson has been about improving my picker.

Let me explain. Sometimes I lack confidence and wonder if I will be lovable if I reveal my truest, fullest personality to another human. Am I too much? When I lack confidence, I can be needy. I seek external validation. I may choose to have a relationship with a person who is not emotionally available. Sometimes I give my power to those people. I waste my energy trying to get them to be the person I want them to be instead of honoring them where they are.

*Dear Big Love,*
*Please give me the clarity and confidence to choose people who are available to be in a relationship with me. Also help me to take responsibility for validating myself and to accept people where they are.*

# 22I

## CLEANING UP COMMUNICATION
## EXPLAIN + DEFEND AND EDITING

*I was raised by well-meaning,* loving, conservative midwestern parents. Messages that were intentionally conveyed to me were honesty, kindness, education, hard work, ambition, perseverance, loyalty, and a sense of humor. Messages that were unintentionally modeled for me included: perfectionism with extreme importance on thinness; impression management; criticism; judgment; sarcasm; out-of-balance other-orientedness; and people-pleasing. Without a doubt I believe my parents did the absolute best they could, and they did an outstanding job.

Although I have many memories of laughing and feeling supported and loved, I don't remember a lot of authentic conversations. Maybe that's why I crave intimate relationships so much. I remember always wanting to just say how I really felt and eat the amount of food I wanted to eat and my mother, mortified, would shhh me or remind me, "A lady doesn't talk like that." Or "that is the portion size a boy or a man would eat!" I know now she was just passing along what was modeled to her by her mother, and so on. I'm at peace with my mom, grateful for all the love she gave me.

Thanks to my upbringing, I have internalized my parents' intended messages and have a strong moral foundation and I am teachable. I look good on paper and I look good on the outside. However, in my 20s, I recognized my communication skills needed work. Due to disordered eating and body dysmorphia that began in grade school, my communication skills stopped at about age 10. I began catching up at around age 26. It is an ongoing loving process.

One thing I've acquired is the ability to edit. I no longer need to tell you EVERY detail when you ask how I am doing today. I call it "explain + defend." I exaggerate to prove my point, but frequently I used to explain and defend every move I made because I thought I had to defend my very existence. Nowadays, when I notice myself explaining and defending, it is a signal to me that I'm giving away my power.

Dear God,
Thanks for the ability to edit what comes out of my mouth right in the moment most of the time. And help me remember it's okay to clean things up after the fact if I forget.

# 222

## AGING FEARS

*Recently my friend Cordelia* (80) experienced weeks of pain and spasming in her back, legs, and neck. She completed an extensive writing workshop where she took inventory of her life, her behaviors, thoughts, and feelings. In the workshop, her fear of aging became apparent. She shared some of her fears with me:

- Afraid her feet would be cold at night with no one to bring her socks.

- She would be unlovable because of unchecked chin hairs.

- She would be unlovable because of what her body looked like (she'd had a mastectomy).

- She would be discounted because her body looked old.

- She would be unloved for being old.

- She would simply be killed because she is considered old and useless.

- She would experience intolerable pain.

Most women would not think these things about other women, yet how many of us think these things about ourselves?

The day she shared the fears with me, she awoke pain-free for the first time in weeks. Looking inward at fears can be a powerful, healing experience.

*Dear Big Love,*
*Please give me the willingness to let go of beliefs that no longer serve me.*

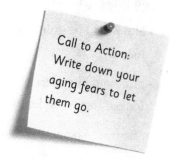

Call to Action:
Write down your aging fears to let them go.

# 223

## Try Something New: Curling Wand Your Hair

*We've been all through my hair inventory:* naturally frizzy/curly hair to flat-ironing and even chemical straightening. The struggle with frizz is real. Fifteen years ago, I learned my hair could be chemically straightened and I have never looked back. Some days I ponder whether I could have entirely avoided my years of self-esteem issues and subsequent disordered eating had I discovered chemical straightening in my teens instead of in my 40s. It is that significant. Thank you, Leela Fuentes!

Having said that, I never thought I would see the day that I got tired of straight hair. But after 12 years of having stick-straight hair, it happened. I was scrolling though social media, looking for God, and I saw a video ad for a curling wand. Completely mesmerized, I watched the entire 45-minute demonstration. There was way too much chitchat, but still I was spellbound. It looked easy. Could I do it? The standard negative self-talk-contempt-prior-to-investigation ensued. These are the things my head says every time I contemplate trying something new. This is why I avoid trying something new.

- I won't be good at it.

- What if I can't figure out how to hold it and I burn myself?

- What if I can't master it?

- What if I look ridiculous and no one tells me?

- What if I hold the wand in place too long and burn off a chunk of my hair like they do on sitcoms?

> Call to Action:
> Name something new you would like to try. Give yourself permission not to be an expert. Now go and try whatever it is you gave a name to!

I bought the wand. I wasn't an expert at first, but I practiced, and I got better! And I didn't care what people thought about how I looked! But a lot of my friends have asked me to curl their hair. And I did burn my fingers a couple of times in the beginning, but then I got the hang of it. And so far, I've not burned any chunks off.

I freakin' love curling my hair now!

# 224

## TRY SOMETHING NEW: MAKEUP APPLICATION AT SEPHORA

*One day I got together for coffee* with my friend Cordelia (50). Her eye makeup was amazing. She had that cool, smokey-eye thing happening. But it wasn't over the top. It was subtle, yet pronounced. I couldn't stop staring. I asked her how she learned to do her makeup like that. "Yasmine at Sephora taught me." Within two weeks, I had an appointment with Yasmine. I had known I needed a makeup update, but was unsure where to turn. Given my age, I was worried that I'd look like a middle-aged woman desperately and unsuccessfully trying to recapture her youth.

The day of the appointment arrived. Fears arose:

- What if I can't replicate what she does?
- What if I can't figure out how to apply the liner and it smears?
- What if I can't master it?

- What if I look ridiculous and I'm posted on social media as a laughingstock as old woman tragically trying but failing to look young again?

- What if I poke my eye with one of the tools?

Despite my loud self-talk, I went. I didn't nail it immediately, but I let that be okay. I did it anyway. I practiced every day. My skills improved.

I love my makeup today!

Reflection:
I give myself permission to try new things and not concern myself with having to be an expert at everything. I keep reminding myself that "good enough" can be good enough. Being a perfectionist is a heavy burden.

# 225

## EXCUSE ME VS. I'M SORRY

*I consider myself* a recovering people-pleaser who special-
izes in impression management. The older I get, the less
these intimacy-avoiding tactics appeal to me or work for
me. They simply stopped working for me. But if I want to
stop a behavior, I do best when I replace the behavior with
another healthier one. One example is saying "I'm sorry."
I used to go around apologizing for everything. Basically,
I might as well have just worn a sign that said, "I am sorry
that I am not everything you want me to be." Now I make a
conscientious effort not to say
"I'm sorry" but instead replace
it with "excuse me" whenever
possible. This sounded so
strange to me at first, but it
has really grown on me.

Reflection:
I ask for God's help to remind
me that I do not need to apologize for my existence. This is
a limiting belief that no longer
serves me. TWBD.

# 226

## EXPLETIVES & F-BOMBS vs. COMPASSION

*I was at the Target intersection today* and saw a guy with a dog on one corner waiting for his green light. His dog did his business, the light changed, and the two entered the crosswalk, seemingly without a care in the world. "WTF!" my head said. I rolled down my car window as I began mentally rehearsing what I would scream at him. My lines included various expletives, including body parts and F-bombs.

Suddenly I stopped myself. Wait. What would compassion look like here? I don't know what his world looks like right now. If I am so into shaming

Dear God,
Help me remember I do not know where another person is coming from. Furthermore, the amount I judge another is the same amount I am judging myself. Help me to calm my own nervous system today.

this guy, what must my stress level be right now? Is there something in me I need to look at right now? That's probably the best he can do. I rolled up my window and drove on.

Call to Action:
Next time you are tempted to judge someone, notice what is being triggered in you that you may be avoiding by focusing on another person's actions.

# 227
## MIND-BODY WALKING

*I am an anxious person.* One of my favorite self-calming activities is what I call "mind-body walking." I walk almost daily, even if only for 10 minutes at a time. Often, I tend to walk mindlessly, not being at all planted where my feet are. When I just mindlessly walk, I am not in the present and I miss out on life. When I participate in mind-body walking, I am experiencing the present moment and get much more out of it.

1. Breath Awareness: Breathe in through your nose; breathe out through your mouth. Try different breath patterns/step combinations such as: Breathe in for 4 steps, hold the breath in for 4 more steps, then exhale for 6 steps.

2. Lift + Separate: Think of your nipples lifting and separating, like the old Playtex bra commercials in the 1960s.

3. Squeeze the Grape: Imagine having a grape in your navel and gently activate your abdominal muscles to prevent the grape from falling out.

4. Supermodel: Swivel your hips as a supermodel would. Walk like you are all that. Because you ARE!

I like to consciously challenge myself by combining all four body "activities." I start with my breath awareness then add the lift + separate, squeeze, and swivel. This is a great mind body exercise to keep in my toolbox.

Dear Nature,
Thank You for ideas about how to calm my nervous system. Thank You for ways to stay close to You.

Call to Action:
Try one breath pattern of mind-body walking today with the option of doing a second breath pattern. Give yourself bonus points for looking a passerby in the eyes as you do this. And give yourself double bonus points for holding position #2 above as you look the passerby in the eye.

# 228

## REALISTIC EXPECTATIONS – YOUR TIMING IS PERFECT: COVID-19

*As I write this entry,* we are about six weeks into global shelter-in-place. For me, making sense of and coping with the pandemic has shone a bright light on some of my lifelong learned behaviors. Thank You, God, for the opportunity to grow ... again. Gratitude leads to acceptance.

The behavior I am referring to is believing the lie my head tells me that I am perpetually behind schedule and need to hurry up. Every time I believe this lie, it creates super-sized doses of cortisol in my system. It destroys my serotonin. I don't want to live like this. This mentality separates me from the God of my understanding and separates me from people I love. Maybe it's a sign that this behavior has outlived its usefulness for me, and I am ready to let go of it.

Dear God,

Help me be willing to let go of old behaviors that no longer serve me. So far, I have been unable to stop believing the lies in my head. Staying in touch with You is my only hope of changing. Your to-do list is the only one that matters. Help me remember:

- My timing is perfect.
- It is okay to stop when my body feels tired.
- What I accomplish today is just the right amount.
- I am enough today.
- I have enough today.
- I desire to be a human being, not a human-doing.
- There are no police coming to monitor the completion of today's to-do list.

Call to Action:

Think of a behavior that has outlived its usefulness. Now write it down and then write the opposite five times. Maybe you have more than one that needs to be addressed, so do this exercise again.

# 229

## NEGATE UNHEALTHY SELF-TALK

*Some mornings* my negative self-talk (NST) is through the roof. This happens a lot on Mondays. Today is one of those days. The CV/CV writing exercise is an extremely helpful tool on days like this.

> *My Critical Voice:*
> *Dear Sally,*
> *Don't even bother to shower today. You shouldn't teach that class at noon. You are tired. Your back hurts. You are a phony. No one wants to hear what you have to say today. You are not good enough. You are too old. You are so far behind on everything. Your house is so cluttered. How can you live like that? You will never accomplish anything, and you are a failure and will be forever. Just give up.*

*My Compassionate Voice:*

*Dear Sally-Girl,*

*Please don't listen to CV. It tells all lies. Showering is a great place to start today and I am so glad you did. Showering is footwork that means you have faith in Love. I cannot wait until you teach your class today. Think about someone else in the class who might be having the same NST as you, and your words will help get them through it. I know you are tired, so how about a 10-minute horizontal unplug before class? That might also relax your back. You are good enough as is. You are real. Your authenticity is what makes you attractive. I love you no matter what your house looks like. You are a success in My eyes every time you suit up and show up for the day and act as if you are lovable. These feelings will pass. Persevere. I am so proud of you. Award!*

*Always remember, God loves you so much He can't take His eyes off you!*

Call to Action:
Maybe there is a critical voice with a bullhorn in your head today. Be willing to try the CV/CV writing exercise today.

# 230

## Faith in the Absence of External Feedback: Career Pivot with COVID-19

*Super-bad negative self-talk today* says don't even shower or show up. I need to ignore the NST that tells me not to bother even getting up today because I am not good enough in any way.

It was a really hard day to live in my head. All day long, my head was saying I'm not good enough. I tried writing CV/CV, I tried praying, I made phone calls to multiple friends. Still, the mean voices continued. I have recently pivoted from teaching classes in person to teaching classes online. Before class, in an effort to quiet the mean negative self-talk in my head, I even prayed for each individual participant who would be coming to the class.

I've learned with experience that when I'm afraid to walk through something and yet I do it anyway, the resulting experience is often euphoria. Today that was not the case. Four hours after the class had ended, the NST was still going like matcha tea on steroids. The uncomfortable feelings were almost debilitating. As uncomfortable as it was, I resolved to sit through the unpleasant feelings, trusting they would pass.

At 6:00 p.m. I received a text from one of the participants out of the blue. In the text, she raved about how much she had gotten out of my class today. I burst into tears. Finally, the negative self-talk lifted.

I am noticing without judgment that no matter how hard I strive to validate myself from within, as a teacher, I still sometimes expect and crave external feedback. I need to be able to physically touch people. I need to be able to see a 3D version of them, which is not possible with video communication. I call it visceral feedback. The important lesson here is that no matter what lies my head tells me, I must continue to persevere toward the thing that makes my heart sing. To persevere toward the message I feel called to share with the world.

Dear God,
Please help me strengthen my internal validation muscle and my faith in You. Make Your comforting presence evident to me as I walk through new life skills and carry out Your will for my Big Amazing Life.

# 231

## Food Prep - Crockpot Chicken

*One of the ways* to boost the immune system is through choosing self-loving foods and amounts. Being a former volume + emotional eater, it's important for me to have nutritional foods readily available in my kitchen, especially during times when emotions are present (which is basically most of the time). One technique that helps me is pre-planning some of the food groups, so they are already ready when I need fuel to live my Big Amazing Life. I have found that discipline leads to happiness and spontaneity leads to chaos.

Prepping a whole chicken for the crockpot is one of my favorite things to do!

*Dear God,*
*Food prep takes a lot of time! Is it worth it?*
*Am I worth it?*
*Love, Sally*

*Dear Sally-Girl,*

*Yes, it does take time, and no one taught you this skill growing up. You are the mom of you now and you are DEFINITELY worth self-loving actions such as food prep. I am so enormously proud of you.*

Call to Action:
Google a recipe
for something and
get prepping.

# 232
## Relationship with Social Media Since COVID-19

*By the time you are reading this,* I pray we have happily and safely returned to global social closeness. However, I bring it up because the topic is relevant, regardless. Perhaps you could say I have social media FOMO (Fear of Missing Out). Before shelter-in-place, I would say I could take it or leave it if you asked me about my relationship with social media. But with the advent of the pandemic, I suddenly find myself checking it a few times per hour or more. I even wake up in the middle of the night and check it. I don't know whether I'm looking for God in there, or Mom, or approval, or love, or a sign that everything will be okay. It's probably a little of each of those things. But this behavior doesn't serve me. It revs up my nervous system and robs me of peace.

Unlike any time in our lifetime, I think we all are preoccupied with issues such as the pandemic and moment-to-moment updates, the Black Lives Matter movement, an extraordinarily divisive presidential campaign and so much more.

I want to challenge myself to refrain from social media on any device for a consecutive 2-hour period, minimum of four days a week. I'm not sure I can do it, but it might save my sanity. If all goes well, I will lengthen the time.

Dear God,
Help me remember to come to You as my source of peace.

Call to Action:
Embrace a 2-hour unplug challenge. Smart phones are off limits! Computer use for writing, research or work-related emails are permissible (ebooks too). No reading online newspapers or shopping. Choose a time block—morning, afternoon, or evening—and stick with that period each day. Unplugging from technology can be a good thing. You may decide to incorporate it into your life!

# 233

## Permission to Take a Break

*I tend to be a little black and white.* As I age, I've noticed this tendency has increased. I find that when engaged in anything, if my mind or body feels tired, I ignore this feeling and tell myself I must "power" through without a break because if I stop to rest, I won't be able to muster the energy to resume later. This mentality leads to fatigue, stress, and inability to fall asleep at night.

Part of the reason for this mentality is the fact that my energy level and stamina are

Dear God,
Remind me to trust You. To trust that if I stop an activity to rest, I will be able to resume the activity with renewed energy. Also remind me to accept that whatever I can accomplish on any given task is the right amount for that day. To know that if I don't end up resuming a desired goal, it means my nervous system has completed enough for that day. Help me let go of my need to prove myself. I am lovable just as I am today.

simply not what they were ten years ago. At some level, I fear I will be deemed obsolete as a human being if I cannot "keep up" with 20-year-old women.

Call to Action:
How does your body signal you that you have done enough? Do your eyes sting a little? Add eye drops if needed. Does your chest feel tight? Do a breathing exercise. Do your joints ache? Go on a short walk. Be willing to listen to your body and heed any negative signals. Give yourself permission to take a break. Maybe reading a good book or taking a nap is in order!

# 234

## Ten-Minute Vitamin D Walking Challenge

*I engage in moderate amounts of exercise* to prevent disease, avoid sarcopenia (muscle loss with aging), improve posture + flexibility, stay mobile, sleep better, and minimize depression. Thirty years ago, these were not my reasons for exercising. I exercised excessively because I thought I was counteracting my bouts of unbridled eating to control my weight. This never worked and kept me on edge, never sure when the next episode of eating with wild abandon would occur. I describe this as a bulimic exercising mindset.

I consider myself a former exercise bulimic. Through my relationship with a being greater than myself, I have recovered from the destructive mindset that tells me I must participate in excessive exercise to control my weight. Also, I have learned that the excessive exercise I used to do was yet another way to avoid feeling my feelings.

Today, my exercise routine is much more balanced. I still sometimes overeat or choose non-nutritional foods, but I forgive myself. As a result, I eat with wild abandon less often and the amount of food I eat is much less. I have learned the secret: When I want to volume-eat, it is because I am trying to stuff down a feeling. The sooner I recognize this and stop to identify and sit with the feeling, the sooner the urge passes, and I can get on with my Big Amazing Life. And exercise has taken its proper place in my life.

Dear God,
Remind me to trust You. Give me the willingness to stop and identify my feelings first when the refrigerator calls my name. Help me achieve the appropriate balance between eating and movement. Give me the ability to exercise for the right reason.

Call to Action:
Take a 10-minute Vitamin D walk today and call it good enough. If you're just hitting your stride, add another 10 minutes!

# 235

## DEALING WITH DEPRESSION – WHO, ME?

*Sometimes I struggle with mild depression.* Often, I don't recognize it because it is subtle. I guess I expect there would be a big sign floating over my head, saying, "See Depression Below" when I am depressed. Of course, that's not the case. Some of the signs I'm depressed are as follows: I won't want to make my bed because "what's the point, I'll just be messing it up again tonight." I will wear the same outfit a few days in a row. I keep washing it every day, but then just wear it again. That's normal, right? I think somehow, I believe this comforts me when I feel like the rest of my life is out of control and the unpredictability of life is too uncomfortable for me.

Once I recognize signs like these, I draw inspiration from one of many beloved mentors in my life. Dr. Patricia Allen, known as Pat Allen, says, "The way out of a negative feeling is a positive decision followed by action." Just for today, I can make a positive decision to make my bed or wear a different outfit and act on that decision.

Dear Universe,
Please guide me to keep in fit mental condition. Whatever that looks like, give me the willingness to get help if necessary.

Call to Action:
Is there a chance you are depressed? If so, make a positive decision to get help. Then get help. Talk with your healthcare provider.

# 236

## SIGNS OF STRESS &
## FEAR OF BECOMING OBSOLETE

*Like my experience with depression,* I tend to be stressed at times and not realize it. There is no "Stress Case Below!" sign floating over my head to alert me. Yesterday my son joined me on a social-distancing permittable dog walk in our local park. There were more people there than usual, and we carefully navigated ourselves and our active dog to keep the required distance between us and passersby. A family with a large dog approached, with only their toddler holding the dog leash. I called out, "Are you planning to put your dog on a leash?"

"He is on a leash." Just then the toddler dropped the leash, rendering the dog completely free. Irritated, I countered something back. I felt like it was an okay thing to say, but my son later pointed out my tone was harsh. They countered back. Eventually an adult took hold of the leash, but not until we had to circumnavigate way off the path to keep a safe distance from them.

As we walked on, I kept grumbling angrily to my son, "Can you believe people like that?" My son's frankness made me even more frustrated. Then I was mad at him on top of that. We walked home in awkward silence. After thinking more about it, I realized the presence of the dog and all the people stressed me out. My tone probably was more critical and harsher than the situation called for. I decided to talk to my son and apologize for letting my anger come out sideways towards him. He was only sharing his honest opinion. Why was this so difficult for me?

Because, I reasoned, if I was being too abrupt, I was not perfect. And if I'm imperfect, maybe I'm unlovable. Maybe I had become obsolete in my son's eyes ... in everyone's eyes. Thank goodness I have learned communication tools to use to

Dear God,
Thank You for giving me the willingness to talk things out with my friends and loved ones, even when I feel silly admitting the way my brain works. I know it is worth the extra effort to stay current in all my relationships.

check things out with the people in my life. We talked it all out. It really had nothing to do with my son and everything to do with my own negative self-talk.

Call to Action:
Think back to an uncomfortable interaction that has taken place between you and someone in your life that you'd like to revisit after the fact. Seek that person out and make amends. There is no statute of limitations on staying current. You are so not obsolete because you are imperfect. Your imperfections make you more lovable.

# 237

## SUNDAYS DURING COVID-19: UNSTRUCTURED TIME ON STEROIDS

*My friend Cordelia* (79) called me one day, struggling with lies her head was telling her. It was Sunday, and Sundays can be challenging because my head is on overtime trying to get me to judge myself. Sunday and shelter-in-place combined can be a lethal combination. Cordelia had been studying the behaviors of external sources such as TV commercials, and social media (becasue that's realistic—NOT). Enough said.

In short, her head was telling her she was falling short as a human being. Her schedule was falling behind. She wasn't getting out at all and she kind of enjoyed the isolation. She had blown off her to-do list. She felt guilty and judgmental about herself. You would think from the disdain in her voice that lethargy was a crime.

We talked about the fact that we are all doing the pandemic and any given season of life the best we know how.

And even then, every day may look completely different from the day before.

Dear Universe,
Please help me remember to live and let live without judgment of myself or others.

Call to Action:
If you are judging yourself or another about anything, let that "anything" go.

# 238

## SELF-TALK MATTERS

*There are some words I try to use as little as possible.* One of those words is the F-word. You may be surprised that I am referring to "fat." This word has a bad connotation for me. Growing up in a family that used this word to judge others had a significant impact on me. My parents never directly called me fat, but they might as well have because I saw the look on their faces and heard the tone in their voices when they used the label to judge a passerby on the street with hushed tones of disdain. For many years, I used this word to describe myself with that same contempt and disdain.

One of the living amends I have made to myself for over 30 years is not to use the F-word to describe myself or others. In fact, when I talk about myself to my son, I am careful only to refer to my body as something I love dearly. I have also raised him to have the same respect for his body and the bodies of others.

Call to Action:

Are there any "F-words" in your vocabulary that you would like to eliminate to make amends to yourself? Be aware of what kind of message you are modeling to your children about your body image, and therefore, their body image. Write down three positive things about your body image in describing yourself.

# 239
## DOING ENOUGH

*Like many of us,* I am in the midst of pivoting my business and my brand to meet the needs of today's culture. Pandemic or not, pivoting calls for radical open-mindedness, courage, and perseverance during a crazy self-talk roller coaster of euphoria and self-doubt. On any given day, so many thoughts run through my head. Am I doing enough? Will I successfully pivot? How will I know? When will I know? Will I make enough money to support myself? Am I a joke? Am I too late?

To quiet these thoughts, I typically employ the CV/CV writing exercise to find the truth and quiet the ridiculous lies my head tells me.

*My Critical Voice:*
*Dear Sally,*
*You are way behind. You are too late. You will not get where you want to be by the time you need to be there*

and thus all your efforts are in vain and you are a loser. Give up. Just eat. Hurry up. You need to do more. Faster. Work harder. Don't rest. It is not enough.

My Compassionate Voice:

Dear Sally-Girl,

Look at you! I am so proud of you. How brave are you? You are right on schedule in every way. Please stop and rest when you are tired. It is okay that you don't have as much energy as your 19-year-old son. Please stop comparing yourself to anyone but you. You compared to you … is a miracle! Keep up a realistic pace for you. You just need to have courage and do the footwork. You know this is what you've wanted to do for years and now is your time to do it. It's undeniable. You are exactly right in every way and I love you so much.

Always remember, God loves you so much He can't take His eyes off you!

Call to Action:
Write down any voices in your head that you need to stop listening to. Now describe at least one way you will go about eliminating each negative voice from your thoughts. Empower yourself to seek out a mental health provider for help/guidance.

# 240
## ROASTED EGGPLANT

*I love to eat.* I embrace that. I am a former volume eater. I embrace that as well. I frequently look up new ways to prepare foods, especially vegetables, to avoid getting in a rut with my food. One new favorite recipe I found was roasted eggplant. It is easy, delicious, and looks fancy!

## Sylvia Fountaine's Roasted Eggplant
Ingredients

> 1 globe eggplant (about 1–1 ⅛lb.)
>
> 1 ½ tablespoons olive oil
>
> 1 tablespoon zataar spice mix (see notes for substitution)
>
> ¼ teaspoon salt, more to taste
>
> 1 fat garlic clove

Served with:

2 cups cooked rice or grains (freekeh, farro, quinoa)

1–2 cups fresh chopped veggies: tomato, cucumber, radish, grated carrot, or beets

Your choice of tahini sauce, plain yogurt, or tzatziki

Other options: Italian parsley, kalamata olives, Aleppo chili flakes, feta, or goat cheese crumbles

Instructions

Preheat oven to 400F

Slice eggplant in half, then slice deeply at a diagonal at one-inch intervals; i.e., "crosshatching." Be careful not to cut through skin.

Season each side with ⅛ teaspoon kosher salt, sprinkling it into the slices if possible.

Mix oil, spices, garlic together in a bowl to make a paste. Brush or spoon the entire contents over the eggplant and place on a sheet pan in the oven and bake for 1 hour, rotating halfway through. After an hour, pierce with a fork and if they are very tender and juicy, they are done. Bigger eggplants may take longer.

When the eggplant is done, assemble the plates, topping warm rice or grain with the roasted eggplant, then surround with fresh veggies and drizzle with tahini, yogurt, or tzatziki – or you could simply eat as is. Add olives or cheese if you wish. Sprinkle with fresh Italian parsley. Enjoy!

*Notes:* If you don't have zataar– then use a substitution of: ½ teaspoon cumin, ½ teaspoon coriander, 1 teaspoon sumac (and if you don't have sumac, sub 1 teaspoon lemon zest, or finely chopped preserved lemon), ½ teaspoon dried oregano or thyme, ½ teaspoon sesame seeds, and a pinch salt.

Dear God,
Thank You for giving me the willingness to try new foods. I am worth the time and effort.

Call to Action:
Find a new recipe today and prepare it.

# 241

## TAKE A SHOWER AND PUT ON REAL PANTS: COVID-19

*These are unprecedented times.* People are scared about things they can't control. Today more than ever, times are uncertain. Here's the thing, pandemic or not, these are still unprecedented times. There are scary things in life you can't control. Times are always uncertain.

A global pandemic is rather like the Universe saying: *Hey, you know that control you thought you had? That's always been an illusion.* Having established that in a huge way, what are you going to do with the rest of your Big Amazing Life … from today on?

Dear God,
Give me the faith to take a shower and put on real pants today and leave the rest to You. Let my thinking be void of criticism and full of open-mindedness about Your will for me today. You are my employer. Use me in a powerful way today. How can I be of service?

Call to Action:
Yes, this is scary. Yes, things are uncertain. Write down what you want to do with your Big Amazing Life.

# 242

## Healing From Diet Mentality: Moderation in Food, Exercise, Self-Talk

*I just saw yet another advertisement* for an over-the-counter antiaging supplement and felt compelled to talk about it. This supplement promised amazing focus, energy, alertness, and mood enhancement! As someone who's worked in the fitness and wellness industry for over 25 years, I've frequently heard claims such as this, as well as claims about diets, shots, pills, and prescription meds, and every combination thereof. A few of these products may prove effective for some people for a finite period, but many of them never work at all.

It has been my experience—both professionally and personally—that whether these products' claims are true or not, one crucial component of the equation is being overlooked completely. The missing component is emotional health and well-being. People want the quick fix. Some people are dissatisfied with their weight and/or their body, and believe if they could just lose weight, they would be happy forever. I call that "diet mentality."

Other people experience chronic physical pain and believe if they could just find the right medication, their pain would cease. I call that "easier, softer way mentality." I have found that many people with "diet mentality" and "easier, softer way mentality" have one thing in common: they avoid identifying uncomfortable emotions and they avoid seeing those emotions through to resolution. In short, for whatever reason, they don't want to address their own personal development. Instead they stay distracted perpetually as they search for what they think will bring happiness through diets, supplements, and pain meds rather than looking within. This state of mind is often accompanied by one or more of the following thought patterns:

- negative self-talk

- negative body image

- low self-esteem

- fear of failure/success that prohibits them from reaching their full potential in life

Sure, when I began my weight loss journey over 30 years ago, I had diet mentality. I wanted the quick fix, too. After six years of repeated failed dieting attempts, I finally resigned from the debate. Through outside help and journal writing, I committed to addressing the emotional and personal development pieces as needed on a consistent basis.

Over time, I developed a series of writing exercises that enabled me to identify feelings and walk through them. With the emotional and spiritual framework in place, the physical and intellectual components fell naturally into place as well. Over the course of slightly more than one year, I lost about 35 pounds. I have kept the weight off through pregnancy, parenting, life's hardships, menopause, and then some. One of the ways I've maintained my weight loss for over three decades is by staying current with emotional health and well-being through writing.

This process has allowed me to cultivate meaningful relationships in every area of my life.

This process has freed me up to thrive professionally as I share this message with others.

This technique has given me freedom to live a joyful, healthy life without diets, supplements, or pain meds.

Dear God,
Thank You for these awarenesses that have given me the freedom to flourish physically, intellectually, emotionally, and spiritually in a moderate-sized body with age-appropriate exercise for over 30 years, through menopause and beyond.

Call to Action:
- Are you tired of quick fixes that don't work?
- Are you ready to get thin between the ears and flourish?
- Are you ready to get out of "diet mentality" and "easier, softer way mentality" and reach your true potential?

Up to this point in my journaling, I've shared lots of tools and techniques in my toolbox. Many I created to help me with a concern. Dessert Day once a week was created to keep my eating expectations realistic.

Create your own unique tool to adhere to or borrow mine so you, too, can achieve moderation in eating, exercise, and self-talk.

# 243

## Train of Thought

*For the last hour* I have been trying unsuccessfully to watch a 13-minute motivational video. This is pretty much my standard scenario. During that time, my distractions included:

- Changing passwords
- Scheduling phone appointment with computer guy
- Scheduling an appointment with the QuickBooks guy
- Attempting to sign up for continuing education for fitness
- Marketing person wanting me to proofread copy
- Banker requesting pdf file that was stored on a flash drive in the fireproof box
- Son wanting to talk about his completed linear analysis midterm
- Barking dog

By now I have pretty much forgotten what my intended activity was.

One of my primary aging challenges has been that everything takes much longer than it used to, and it is much harder to stay focused. But experience tells me that beating myself up has never helped any situation.

*Dear Big Love,*
*Please help me strike a balance between staying focused and going with the flow.*
*Love, Sally*

*Dear Sally-Girl,*
*Whatever you accomplish today is just the right amount. You are right on schedule and right where you are supposed to be. There is no hurry. All is well.*
*Love, Big Love*

# 244

## DONE WITH PEOPLE-PLEASING & COMPULSIVE DOING

*Before shelter-in-place,* one of the ways I avoided feelings was to be compulsively busy. I was always on top of it. By "it," I mean everything. I returned phone calls quickly. I think my voicemail had only ever been full twice in 20 years. I usually entered my receipts into QuickBooks the same day. I took immense pride in my efficiency. I derived much of my sense of self-worth from being efficient. In some ways, efficiency and completion of my massive to-do list were my higher power.

During the first month of shelter-in-place, something inside me changed. A new sense of purpose came over me. I didn't know where it came from, but I just knew it happened; it was unmistakable. A voice said, "Now is the time." I was laid off from one job and the other job violated the social-distancing policy and most of my clients opted to put their sessions with me on hold rather than deal with virtual sessions. There were no more excuses. I knew that meant now was the time to act on some long-held goals I had been pushing aside for more years than I wanted to admit. I knew if I didn't act now, during shelter-in-place, I would never act.

I got to work. ... I went the entire month without entering any receipts. I experienced anxiety over this lack of efficiency, but something inside me changed. I was lucky if I responded to voicemail messages within 76 hours. My voicemail was almost continually full. The pain of not accomplishing these goals became more painful than letting go of compulsive doing. Still, I am jonesing (having a strong desire or craving) for some list completion, don't get me wrong. And the daily fear I am walking through in this process is almost paralyzing, almost ... but not enough to stop. My faith in myself is through the roof and there's no stopping me now. There is no fear that is bad enough to keep me from sharing my message with the world. I am finished playing small.

Dear God,
Please keep me on track. Use me in a powerful way.

# 245

## LIIT (Low-Intensity Interval Training): the HIIT-Solution for Weekly Chore Buildup

*A good six weeks* into the COVID-19 shelter-in-place, and I still flounder some days to find a rhythm. Clients and friends tell me they are experiencing the same thing.

My friend Cordelia (39) noticed with anxiety that a huge pile of paperwork had accumulated in her office. This was not the norm for her. On top of that, other weekly tasks she typically enjoyed—such as cooking, laundry, brushing her dogs, returning emails and voicemails—had built up as well. The fact that she was behind on things she enjoyed doing compounded her stress level and caused an uncomfortable paralysis she was unaccustomed to.

She also noticed old behaviors resurfacing, such as mindless eating. Having lost over 60 pounds through mindful eating, the mindless eating really got her attention. Concerned, she pondered what to do. The administrative task seemed unusually daunting to her. She felt she should just buckle down and plow through it in one sitting. She simply couldn't bring herself to begin.

She came up with a system. She adopted an interval system whereby she set a timer and worked 30 minutes on the dreaded paperwork. Next, she pivoted to laundry, which to her was a break compared to the paperwork. Then she did food prep for 30 minutes, followed by 30 more minutes of the paperwork. And so it went for a good part of her afternoon. Over the course of three hours, she completed ALL her paperwork, her laundry, and her food prep. She felt so good about herself that her eating returned to its former mindful state.

When life circumstances throw a curveball, be open to new ways of handling your former routines. Go with the flow. Think outside the box. Create new neural pathways.

Dear Universe,
Please give me the clarity to be willing and able to stagger tasks I dread—mostly cooking, cleaning, and taxes—with tasks I find more doable.

# 246

## Letting Fear of Criticism Hold Me Back: Thank You, COVID-19

*I have allowed fear of criticism* to hold me back for years. Same story with my perfectionism. In other words, my fear was greater than the pain of my stagnation. Although both have decreased considerably, there is still room for improvement. For some reason, this novel virus has given me a different perspective on both learned behaviors and the willingness to risk criticism like never before.

The global nature of our situation causes me to feel a stronger connection to my fellow humans than I've ever experienced. The connection begets a craving for still deeper connection. Intuition in me knows there is no place for fear or perfectionism in this equation. Hence, this spiritual moment of clarity frees me to risk being more authentic than ever before without fear.

The presence of the pandemic caused an internal mindset shift, making it 51-percent painful to remain stagnant. Once that occurred, although tempting at times, there has been no turning back.

Call to Action:
When remaining stagnant becomes 51-percent painful you will find yourself shedding fears and taking new risks. Write down a fear you have let hold you back. What is one action you can take to walk through that fear?

# 247

## MEMORY, SELF-TALK, & INTIMACY

*I have a memory condition.* There is no permanent cure. The condition is called CRS or Can't Remember S*** (I pretend it stands for stuff, but that requires another asterisk). My CRS is something that has developed in the last ten or so years and coincides roughly with my personal shifting hormone journey. When I first began experiencing CRS, I was devastated. I felt angry. I felt frustrated. I worried I wouldn't be lovable if I was forgetful. I feared I would be judged by others as an old, useless, obsolete person. I especially feared what my son would think of me. That he would be disappointed in me. This may sound extreme, but it is the truth.

Over time I've learned to embrace it and even laugh at it, which is a miracle in and of itself. I finally came to realize that I am not loved because of my performance, but rather because of who I am and how I love myself and others. People I love don't really care if I forget stuff, especially my son. One more time I was reminded that me being me (imperfect) and letting others see that is the actual definition of intimacy (in-to-me-see). It gives gives others permission to be imperfect as well.

Dear God,
Help me remember that expecting perfection from myself and beating myself up for making mistakes has never been a successful technique for "whipping myself into shape." It has never once brought about a change for the better in me.

Call to Action:
Think of a behavior that you've been berating yourself for in hopes of changing it. Are you willing to embrace it instead?

# 248

## Posture, Dog Walks, & Mnemonics

*Besides having the memory issue* I call CRS, I also have another malady which I call ISM. ISM also has no permanent cure.

ISM stands for Incredibly Short Memory. ISM is something I have lived with for over 30 years. ISM is a term I use lovingly to describe my brain's tendency to forget anything or any behavior that is good for me physically, intellectually, emotionally, or spiritually. I have learned to create techniques to help minimize the negative effect ISM has on me.

One example of how ISM symptoms manifest in me involves my posture. We all want good posture, right? Do you think I want a rounded upper back and a forward head that progressively worsens as I age? Of course not. Do you think I want to be one of those people in the grocery story who must use a cart to hold myself up? Although I know I would still be just as lovable if I were, I would most likely be in a lot of pain from that situation. Having said all that, remembering to carry myself with good posture frequently alludes me. Hence, I have found that creating mnemonics is super helpful. A mnemonic is any learning technique that aids information retention or retrieval in the human memory.

One technique I use to combat ISM on posture is what I call the posture/dog-walking technique. While I'm walking my dog, he frequently stops to smell things and mark his territory proudly. Each time he stops for any reason, I take this as a signal that it is time to check my posture. I stand tall and lift my sternum. I lift and separate my chest muscles. I imagine I have a grape in my navel, and I squeeze the grape gently with my abdominal muscles. I breathe in through my nose and breathe out through my mouth. When he is ready, we walk on until the next stop. And that is how I have learned to work around my ISM.

Call to Action:
Do you suffer from ISM? Name one area where you have experienced it. Now create your own mnemonic that you can start using to help your situation.

# 249
## MEDIOCRE OVEN-CLEANING AWARD

*Yesterday I made this amazing banana bread.* Unfortunately, I filled the loaf pan way too full and as the bread baked, the batter spilled out onto the bottom of the oven and burned. The resulting smell was awful, and lingered long after the banana bread was finished. It was so bad I realized I would need to clean the oven. It takes a lot to get me to clean an oven. I don't think I have cleaned my oven since we moved here four years ago. Yes, you know it was really bad. Suffice it to say, it was time.

Given my all-or-nothing mentality, my thoughts defaulted to, "Sally, you must now do a completely thorough oven-cleaning!" I don't even know what that means, but I know it would take at least an hour. I flash back to my mother in the 1970s teaching me to clean the oven. We wore rubber gloves and protective aprons. I remember we had to open all windows and spray the oven with something in an aerosol can, then wait an hour with the oven heated to the lowest possible temperature. The subsequent steps involved massive scrubbing, which massacred your fingernails (hence the gloves) while contorting yourself into strange positions with half your body inside the oven. It would end with my mom lying in bed with a debilitating backache.

Suddenly with great delight, I realized it would be good enough to do a mediocre oven-cleaning! I don't even know if that oven-cleaning aerosol can still exists, but I had neither that nor SOS pads. I cleaned the oven with nothing but my kitchen sponge and called it good. This is what a recovering perfectionist does. I consider this Varsity growth! Malodor gone, sanity restored, problem solved. I even scored a few bonus points because I discarded the sponge when finished and traded up for a brand new sponge.

*Dear Sally-Girl,*
*Mediocre oven-cleaning AWARD!*
*I am so proud of you every time*
*you give yourself permission NOT*
*to be perfect.*
*Love, Big Love*

Call to Action: Identify one thing you can do imperfectly today. Do it ... and give yourself an AWARD!

# 250

## REJOICING IN ALL OF ME

*I describe myself as many things.* Some descriptions I'm prouder of than others. For example, I'm proud to describe myself as quirky. I can easily say I enjoy a dry, *Get Smart/Carol Burnett Show*-type of humor. *Get Smart* was an American comedy TV series that ran from 1965-1970, parodying the secret-agent genre popular in the early 1960s.

I am compassionate. I am creative. The longer I live, the more I realize the importance of embracing all of me ... my perceived strengths and weaknesses. I love the saying, "That which we resist, persists."

I also describe myself as a little too other-oriented. This is a little more difficult to admit. One of the ways this characteristic manifests itself is people-pleasing and what I call "taking people's temperature." I sometimes think I can read minds and know what others are thinking. Consequently, I edit how I interact with them to make them feel at ease and therefore like me more—as if their physical and emotional comfort determines what they think of me, as if their comfort determines my value. As my friend Cordelia says, "Sally, I don't think you have that much power!"

I realize that underlying this belief system is the deeper unrealistic fear that one day it will be determined that I am completely unlovable and will be alone. There it is. It's important to acknowledge that, even though there is still room for improvement here, I have come a long way recovering from this.

This is a behavior that was modeled in my family growing up. Or maybe it wasn't modeled for me and that was just my interpretation of what was modeled. In any event, all that matters is my awareness of the behavior and how I handle myself going forward.

*Dear Sally-Girl,*
*Today I will be here to gently and constantly remind you that you are powerless over people's opinions of you. I will bring just the right people into your day today. Your job is to choose self-loving food groups and portions, strive to seek and do My will, and be only you. Trust that the right people will be in your life today, tomorrow, and always.*
*Love, God*

# 251
## Neuroplasticity, Eating, & Expectations

*This morning I woke up with a bad attitude.* When I feel like this, one might call it "stinkin' thinkin'." The agenda for today includes some tasks I don't enjoy doing. Tasks where I am not the expert; I hate that. Tasks that reduce the amount of time I get to spend doing things I enjoy. Let's call these tasks necessary "adulting" obligations. We all have them. I get that. In short, attitude adjustment is called for. How will I accomplish that? Neuroplasticity, eating, and expectations come to mind. Let me explain.

Science and the plasticity of the brain is fascinating to me. Think of the word malleable. Think capable of change. The notion that the neural pathways—or the connections between and among neurons in the brain—can be changed is exciting. The brain can adapt in response to interaction with the environment. This gives me hope! Neural pathways can be weakened or strengthened ... based on what data we reinforce and what data we stop reinforcing. Whatever we focus on grows stronger.

Originally it was thought by scientists that the brain only had neuroplastic capabilities until we were 25 years of age. Good news! Turns out we are capable of forging new neural pathways our entire lives. All we need to do is get enough sleep, exercise, and continue learning new things. Small price to pay for such an amazing ability. What will I do today to strengthen the appropriate pathways in my brain? Eating and expectations are top priorities.

First, I think about what foods I will fuel my body with. Just for today. I plan nutritional food choices. Thinking ahead about what I will eat helps me avoid spontaneous non-nutritional choices

Call to Action:
Which neural pathways will you strengthen today? It's your choice. Write down what actions you will take and take them! Remember to check that your expectations are realistic.

if I become uncomfortable or stressed. I make a nutrient-dense green smoothie to grab quickly between tasks. Next, I visit my expectations.

As discussed, it's typical for my expectations to be way too high on any given day. For example, when I check my expectations for today, I admit I expect to complete about six hours of work on my current passion project. Having unrealistic expectations is a setup for disappointment and steals my serenity. I adjust that to a more realistic two days.

I'm feeling better already and it's only 8:00 a.m.

# 252

## DEATH OF THE FRIEND'S GRAVEYARD & BIRTH OF NEW NEURAL PATHWAYS

*Another part of me I'd rather keep to myself* is the less-than-mature way I used to view friendships. I was constantly seeking the perfect best friend. The person who fulfilled my companionship needs in every possible way. I wanted someone with my great sense of humor, intelligence, and same hobbies … basically, my clone. Kind of egotistical, right? Although this might be developmentally appropriate for a 12-year-old girl, it became a problematic objective for a maturing woman. To tell you the truth, it never worked well, even at 12. I was constantly disappointed because, of course, that person doesn't and shouldn't be expected to exist. Nevertheless, I "auditioned" countless people for the "job," always disappointed sooner or later. Then I would figuratively throw the person in the "Friend's Graveyard." The Friend's Graveyard is another interpretation of the behavior modeled by my family growing up. As always, it is noteworthy to remind myself not to place blame. The important thing is what I do with the observation going forward. How can I use this as a personal growth opportunity?

I am happy to say, I have made a lot of progress on this. I have figuratively "blocked" the pathway to the Friend's Graveyard. The literal neural pathway in my brain has outlived its usefulness. I have created new neural pathways to replace it using newly acquired intimacy and communication skills.

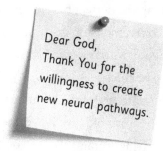

Dear God,
Thank You for the willingness to create new neural pathways.

# 253
## REJOICING IN THE NO

*I've already established* that an awareness of how you feel is easier for me to tune into than the awareness of how I feel. Having established that, there have been times in the past when I neglected to ask a person for what I really wanted. I feared putting the friend/colleague/acquaintance in an uncomfortable position. As crazy as this may sound, I was afraid the other person might also be other-oriented and say yes without wanting to, just to make me happy. Then the person would resent me. So rather than risk all that, I would just skip the request altogether.

For whatever reason, I have tended to gravitate toward people-pleasers in the past because we speak the same language and our flawed communication style was at least familiar. Today, this communication style has outlived its usefulness for me. The overthinking gyrations that underlie people-pleasing can be exhausting! I might have to take a nap just from articulating it.

It is much simpler to just stay in my own hula hoop and ask for what I want. Like many times in life, learning new communication skills proved to be a multistep process. When I began asking for what I wanted, inside I resented people when they gave me a "No."

> *Dear Cordelia,*
> *Why won't you do what I want? My idea is fantastic, and you are stupid not to see that and join me doing what I have asked. That's it. You are so in the Friend's Graveyard.*

Today I ask for what I want and rejoice in the "No" rather than resist it. I may have to do a little writing on paper to get to the rejoicing part, but I get there.

> *Dear Big Love,*
> *Please show me how to give people the dignity of making their own decisions while staying in the relationship and without resenting them for it. While You are at it, please help me discern those relationships that are still appropriate for me on my ever-evolving journey and those I shall lovingly let go.*
> *Love, Sally*

*Dear Sally-Girl,*
*Be ever-patient with the process and with yourself.*
*Something or someone better is always coming.*
*Love, Big Love*

# 254

## Donut Smell Reframing: I Have Choices

*This morning on my walk,* the smell of donuts frying at the local donut shop inhabited my nostrils. It was sublime. A brief conversation in my head ensued. Wouldn't donuts be nice this morning? They taste so wonderful.

Because I have embraced all foods and made peace with my body for over 30 years now, I would experience absolutely no shame if I spontaneously decided to have donuts. In fact, I generally plan one day each month where I do have donuts and it is glorious and shame-free.

Next, I remember the inflammation hangover, stomach upset, and irritability I experience after having eaten high-sugar fried foods. I smile to myself and think: I always have a choice. There are no bad or good foods. Today I gratefully choose not to have donuts because I want my insides to feel good.

I finished feeding the dog and sat down gratefully with my cashews and celery/grapefruit juice, grinning from ear to ear. I always have a choice.

*Dear Big Love,*
*I'm grateful for donuts.*
*I'm grateful for this strong body.*
*I'm grateful for shame-free eating.*
*I'm grateful for choices.*
*Love, Sally*

# 255
## HEALING BREATH

*For years I have dealt with negative self-talk* (NST) in my head. In my early adult life, I became aware of it and the crippling effect it was having on me. In response to the awareness, I developed writing techniques to address it, which have served me well for years.

Recently, my friend Cordelia (40) talked about negative self-talk in a way I had not heard before—or I was just not ready to hear it until yesterday. In any event, she referred to negative self-talk as a form of self-abandonment. Yes! How sad but true is that? For me, it was a moment of clarity, a light-bulb moment. Something resonated for me at the cellular level.

Fascinated, I thought about the concept of self-abandonment on and off all that day. I listened to my body. I realized I can feel self-abandonment as a physiological sensation in my body. The first thing that happens is I notice my head telling me I need to do more, accomplish more, and do it faster. Next, I believe that lie and I feel hopelessly behind and disappointed in myself. Parts of my body tighten, especially my chest. The self-talk is going on and on about the fact that I need to hurry up and complete the XYZ task.

Soon thereafter, I became aware of NST in my head. It was the usual lies about my not performing enough and not being productive enough and not being anything enough. I remembered Cordelia's words and labeled it self-abandonment. This time I tried something new.

I crossed my hands over my heart and took five deep breaths as I said the following five sentences:

*I'm so sorry you're hurting.*
*I'm so sorry you're scared.*
*You are right on schedule.*
*What do you need?*
*How can I help?*

Dear God,
Thank You for my ability to hear the term "self-abandonment" today. Use me in a powerful way to heal from it and help others do the same.

Call to Action:
Is it possible you have abandoned yourself on some level? Be willing to try the reclamation breathing technique.

This technique was extremely calming. And I repeated it each time the NST resurfaced and it was equally calming every time.

# 256

## TRADING HIGH HEELS FOR SNEAKERS

*My friend Cordelia* (50) posted on social media yesterday for the first time in a while. In her post, she said she traded in her high heels for sneakers. After both her sons went away to college in Japan, she, too, moved to Japan. After 25 years, she quit her job in the banking industry. After almost a year in seclusion, she began a different career as an elementary school teacher. She is deliriously happy and fulfilled.

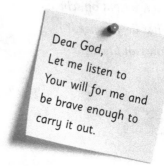

Dear God,
Let me listen to Your will for me and be brave enough to carry it out.

# 257

## The Languages of Fitness

*In my late 20s,* I made radical lifestyle changes on the physical, intellectual, emotional, and spiritual levels. I made peace with my body and I made peace with food. I lost about 35 pounds for the last time, God willing. Having been a yo-yo dieter beginning at age 10, my primary objective was to not only take the weight off, but to keep the weight off long-term. I soon learned that to experience lifelong weight-loss maintenance, my participation needed to be on multiple levels. This was not simply going to be a journey about physical recovery. Yes, my body was now officially "right-sized," but there was so much more to it than the size of my physical body.

As a fitness professional and former bulimic exerciser, I knew all about staying in fit physical condition. What I didn't know was how to stay in fit spiritual condition. Fit emotional condition. Fit intellectual condition. To maintain my new body, I needed all four. I had lost the weight so many times before, only to gain it and even more weight back. This time I was determined to go to any lengths. To do whatever it took. Around the age of 28, I embarked on an entirely new journey which I am still (usually) happily on today at the age of 60. Even through pregnancy at 40, perimenopause and beyond, I remain in what I call a right-sized body and mind.

- A body I can do business with.

- A body I love the hell out of.

- A body that allows me to connect with the people in my life and fulfill my deepest purpose.

Call to Action:
If you desire long-term weight maintenance in a healthy body, be willing to embrace new concepts around your fitness. Write what that would look like on the following levels: physical, intellectual, emotional, and spiritual.

# 258

## PRACTICE MAKES PROGRESS

*I maintain my weight loss* by staying in fit emotional condition. As a child, I ate emotionally because I was never taught that feeling my feelings was healthy, normal, and appropriate. The way I began recovering from emotional eating was to acknowledge I ate emotionally and let it be okay.

To this day I still eat emotionally sometimes, but because of this blanket permission I've given myself, the bouts of unbridled eating are much farther apart, and the quantities consumed are much smaller.

Call to Action: Just for today, try writing down what you plan to eat today.

There is a great tool called "HALT" that helps me reduce the occurrence of emotional eating, so I keep this acronym in my toolbox. HALT stands for "Never get too Hungry, Angry, Lonely, or Tired." Making small daily self-care contracts helps me honor HALT.

# 259

## TAKE BREAKS AGAINST YOUR BETTER JUDGMENT

My head tells me I must press on for hours without a break. I simply cannot stop. If I stop, I will lose my momentum and forget where I was and perhaps never be able to resume whatever task was at hand.

Today is Sunday. "Finally, maybe I can catch up," my head says. Then my friend Cordelia (50) invited us over for a visit. No special reason, just to hang out and chat. Part of me resisted. "Oh no," my head said, "You have so much to do. This was your one chance to finally catch up. You are so behind on everything." I love Cordelia and her family. They have truly mastered the art of socializing. They are down-to-earth, no-BS, real people. Against my better judgment, I accepted their invitation. We sat on their front porch, talking for over an hour.

At first, it almost killed me to be so unproductive. I felt uncomfortable and squirmed in my chair. I silently talked to myself to assuage my discomfort. "It is totally okay. Nothing is expected of us but to listen and talk when spoken to." After a while, I surrendered to the now. I noticed the beautiful weather … the birds singing … the gentle breeze on my arms and face. It was lovely. I came home and got right back to the task I had been working on, feeling completely refreshed. So why do I resist things like this?

Maintaining the "pressing on" at all costs mindset has some severe costs: heart disease and missing out on spending time with people you love, to name a few. Taking a break will refresh and refill your creative well. I promise.

Dear God,
Please help me today with balance. Thank You for people like Cordelia in my life whose lead I can follow. Thank You for speaking to me through people like her.

Call to Action:
Think of a break you could allow yourself to take today. Now take it!

# 260

## No OPF

*I love mnemonics.* I need all the memory aids I can get. Mnemonics engage and challenge my brain while helping me self-care in a varsity way. I also love free food. I am not sure why, but I've always been this way. When I have worked in an office and someone brings in food, I get excited. Even if I had already loosely planned what I would eat for the day, somehow everything would go out the window and unbridled eating was ON! Eventually I realized that unbridled eating or eating with wild abandon usually ended in consumption of non-nutritive foods that gave me a stomachache, acid reflux, painfully inflamed joints, or all of the above.

Out of this realization, the term OPF (other people's food) was coined. In general, I avoid eating OPF. Just because spontaneous brownies cross my path in the office or via a well-meaning neighbor, it doesn't mean that I throw my self-care contract out the window. The other beauty of OPF is I know when I eat OPF, I am probably experiencing a feeling that I am trying to stuff down. Spontaneous eating is my barometer to notify me of this, and that it is time to explore what those feelings are using a writing technique.

Am I saying I never eat junk food? No, of course not. I am saying that I do better when I refrain from bouts of spontaneous eating. I am saying if I am going to choose non-nutritious foods, I do better when they are planned by me. I know how much I love myself by the contracts I am willing to make and keep—thank you, Pat Allen.

If I could eat with wild abandon any time I felt like it without physical, intellectual, emotional, or spiritual consequences, I would be all over that. But until I figure out how to do that, I don't eat OPF. Nothing beats the feeling of walking out of an office party without a food hangover.

Dear God,
Help me remember I always have a choice in the foods I eat. And remind me that I self-care with food so I can show up for my Big Amazing Life.

Call to Action:
Think about situations involving food that continually have a frustrating result for you. Write down a couple of alternatives to OPF that would work for you.

# 261

## BAN NEGATIVE SELF-TALK RATHER THAN FOODS

*Some days I wake up and my self-talk is brutal.* If my body were a radio, my brain would be tuned to KFCK, all bad … all the time. There are several techniques I use to change that channel to KJOY. One of my favorites is to be accountable about my NST to another safe person. Once I say my actual thoughts aloud to another person, it is embarrassing at first because the things my brain tells me are outlandish. Like that my son will soon have dropped out of college, become addicted to drugs, and end up in prison—all because he likes how he looks in a beard. Inevitably it is comical as my whole thought process is revealed. Sometimes when I call my friend Cordelia, she will add to my wild future-tripping, demonstrating she gets me because she does the same thing, and we laugh hysterically. We have a good laugh and just like that, the crazy talk has vanished, and I can keep listening to KJOY for hours to come.

Some people diet endlessly, forever searching in vain for that magic formula to bring them lasting peace, joy, and contentment. Rather than career dieting and banning foods, why not ban negative self-talk by committing to telling another within 24 hours of noticing it?

Dear God
Please give me the willingness to determine the deeper issue behind my endless dieting. Help me be willing to connect with another human in a powerful way.

Call to Action:
Be willing to look beyond finding the "perfect diet" to find joy. Now think about what brings you joy.

# 262

## Right-Sizing Exercise

*Just as it is vital* to right-size my attitude and self-talk, so too is it vital to right-size my attitude about exercise. I exercise for disease prevention and for cardiovascular strength. I exercise to help me sleep, to lift depression, and to combat sarcopenia.

The following are NOT reasons I exercise (or excessively exercise):

- To eat bigger portions and avoid uncomfortable feelings

- To counter a recent episode of binge-eating

- To apologize for my body's appearance

A wise woman taught me that exercise should be like sex. It should feel good and you should like doing it.

Enough said.

Dear God,
Please help me determine my appropriate exercise routine honoring my body without comparing myself to others, especially my 20-year-old self.

# 263

## FLOWING WITH TECHNOLOGY

*The smart phone keyboard is small.* I get really frustrated when I could swear I've hit an "I", but a "U" keeps appearing. It's not unusual for this error to recur several times during one attempted text. Why is it necessary for me to text? Or use a smart phone? Or participate on social media?

When my son was in high school, I knew the time for him to leave the nest was drawing near. His rigorous AP/IB schedule kept him quite busy, but I wanted a way to stay involved in his life in these precious last few years. I decided to read his US history textbook so that we could talk history together. Besides, I enjoy history, and don't remember a thing from my high school history classes.

In my reading about westward expansion in the US in the 1800s, I read about two people who experienced enormous success. Leland Stanford built part of the first transcontinental rail line, even though many objected to railroad expansion. Railroads united the states and brought about huge growth for the nation. John D. Rockefeller developed an oil-refining process to streamline efficient use of oil in a major way.

I marveled at how people like these flourished in the wake of the Civil War. They flourished because they had the foresight to believe that new things had a potential to change the world. It struck me that the reason these people succeeded was because they were open-minded and thought outside the box before that was even a thing.

Yes, the smart phone keyboard is small. I get really frustrated because it is new for me, but I am thankful for the voice microphone capability. Why is it necessary for me to text? Or use a smart phone? Or participate on social media? Then I remember ...

Dear God,
Help me remember to keep an open mind about new technology. Give me the ability to be patient with myself as I learn a new skill. It's never too late.

# 264

## EVERY RELATIONSHIP ENDS

*There are a lot of amazing people in the world* with whom I have had the privilege of being in a relationship. Relationships can be many things: long, short, romantic, platonic, deep, casual, intimate, professional, fun, serious, heartwarming, challenging, healthy, dysfunctional, informative, messy/complicated, loving, painful, interdependent, codependent, family, and any combination thereof. A relationship is not validation of my worth, meaning I do not need to be in a relationship with another human being to prove my lovability.

A wise woman once told me every relationship ends. I really hated to hear that. At the time, I was struggling with a boyfriend breakup. I made the decision to end the relationship with him because it was 51-percent painful. Still, I was miserable because I had thought he was the one. She told me this because she sensed that I was a little too invested in seeking validation from someone outside of me, regardless of the cost, instead of looking within to find that needed piece.

As hard as that was to hear, she was right. Her words still ring true today. When I am repeatedly challenged by a relationship with a person, I go back to my wise friend's words and ask a power greater than myself, "What is the lesson here? Have we gone as far as we can go together? Is it time to let go?"

Dear God,
Please give me knowledge of Your will regarding my relationship with _____. Has this relationship run its course?

Call to Action:
Think of a relationship that might be more than 51-percent painful. Now decide if it would be best to end the relationship for your mental and emotional well-being.

# 265

## WALL OF KINDNESS

*Some relationships don't work out* and can easily be terminated. If a checker at the grocery store pushes my buttons, I can avoid going to his/her line. When my former housecleaners sent me a verbally abusive/shaming text for the second time, I knew it was time to terminate that relationship (even though they were outstanding in every other way).

Then there are other relationships that cannot be terminated, either because it is someone at your work, or it is a family member. Of course, there are various ways to avoid unpleasant interaction with that person. Boundaries can be set, but some people refuse to honor them. When it comes to sharp tongues, mine is like a razor, but I have learned that the price my nervous system pays when I choose to verbally spar with a toxic person is too great. Of course, if my physical or emotional safety is in question, I do not put myself in a situation under any circumstances. But sometimes an unpleasant interaction simply cannot be avoided. This is when I use the wall of kindness. Usually my kindness will dissipate the angry words and frustration of the other person quickly. The person is anticipating retaliatory words, not words of kindness.

The wall of kindness may be self-explanatory, but basically it means that whatever conversation I have with this person in this isolated, unavoidable situation comes from kindness. No matter what the person says, I respond with kindness. It can be extremely challenging, but if accomplished, it is extremely satisfying. The wall of kindness changes me on the cellular level. It changes my chemistry. It increases my compassion. It decreases my proclivity to emotionally eat. Besides, I can always go home and write an MDK letter and say what I really wanted to say!

Call to Action:
Was there a situation today where you could have used the wall of kindness? Now you have this technique in your toolbox to use as the need arises.

There are three important facts I have learned:

1. It is unrealistic to expect to like everyone I meet.

2. A big part of life is about relationships and about getting along with people without judgment.

3. If I am judging you, it means I am most certainly judging me twice as harshly.

It behooves me to make every effort to get along with people … whatever that looks like.

# 266

## PERSEVERANCE: A TENET OF TAEKWON-DO FITS ME

*My 20-year-old son* has been involved in taekwon-do since he was six years old. Taekwon-do is a Korean martial arts practice that teaches self-defense, movement patterns, and board-breaking with hands and feet. Underlying the physical aspect of taekwon-do are five tenets which are stated at the start of each class: courtesy, integrity, perseverance, self-control, and indomitable spirit. The hope is that each student will not only practice these principles in class, but also practice them in their daily lives outside of the martial arts school.

As I've mentioned, when I was 52, I joined my then-12-year-old son in his taekwon-do classes. Of all the tenets, my favorites were always perseverance and indomitable spirit. I know they always say life is not easy, but I guess I never realized how challenging it can be sometimes. Or how hard I must work if I really want to make a difference in the lives of others ... like really hard. So, when things get tough and I want to quit because I am believing negative self-talk lies my head is telling me, I remember standing there in that hideously unflattering white uniform, beside my son, chanting those five tenets. And I was forming an unforgettable bond with my son for life.

Dear God,
Please remind me when something is hard that if it is worth achieving, it is worth the hard work. Like really hard work. And refresh my spirit when I want to give up.

# 267

## Imperfection & Choice Cheat Sheet

*Perfectionism is destructive.* It hurts me and severely limits my ability to be vulnerable with you.

Just for today, I choose not to let my perfectionism distract me from my friendship with you. If you judge me for my imperfections, it was never a friendship anyway.

Just for today, I choose to let things go even if they are done imperfectly. Good enough is just that.

Just for today, I choose to let go of your opinion of me. That doesn't have my name on it.

Just for today, I give myself permission to be nobody but me. Have a mediocre day!

**Call to Action:**
Just for today, choose to let something in your daily routine be imperfectly done. Tell yourself: Good enough is good enough for that task/chore today!

# 268

## KEEP IT SIMPLE

*My friend Cordelia* (35) is a woman of few words. But when she says something, I lean in. Yesterday she summed up her three guidelines for a healthy eating mindset:

- No diets.
- No deadlines.
- No damage control.

*No diets:* I no longer punish myself with dieting. Diets are simply a distraction that keeps me from doing the inner work I need to do to fall in love with myself. Diets will never bring about the self-love I yearn for. Whatever you eat to take the weight off is what you will need to continue to eat to keep the weight off. Diets perpetuate the problem. Eating in moderation is the solution.

*No deadlines:* I no longer subject myself to unrealistic, rigid expectations and time constraints about how fast I must lose how many pounds by what event date.

*No damage control:* There will be times I overeat. When this happens, I no longer require myself to cut back on subsequent meals to "make up for" my earlier bouts of spontaneous eating. Eating is not a moral issue.

Call to Action:
There is no magic. Be willing to go to any lengths to let go of your diet mindset. Do the work to fall in love with yourself. You've got this!

# 269

## MORE WACKY GRATITUDE: ROOF LEAKS & LAYOFFS

*On the morning of December 26, 2019,* I sat up in bed, put my feet on the floor and it was wet. Like really wet. Turns out the heavy rain the night before, coupled with a roof leak, resulted in a puddle on the floor almost twice the size of my bed. Merry Christmas to me!

For those of you who have experienced a major water leak in your home, you know what is involved: the 24-hour restoration guys; the dislocated sleeping arrangements; the very loud fans (shhhhhhhh!); the wall cutting; the insurance people; and the flooring guys. It's an endless parade of workmen. Did I mention the loud fans? For about 21 days? "Thank You, God, for this growth opportunity" was my mantra.

About the end of February, the work was finally completed. About a week later, I was laid off from my dream job after only six months. As are many layoffs, this was completely unanticipated. The timing was about one week before COVID-19 called for shelter-in-place. "Thank You, God, for this growth opportunity."

Sometimes I really don't get God's reasoning or His timing. Usually I feel as if things that happen are not supposed to be happening and God has made a huge mistake. I usually journal to Him just how I feel about His timing and He gets an earful. Yet I also continue to write my wacky gratitude lists throughout this season. Gratitude leads to acceptance. Gratitude and acceptance heal me on the cellular level.

Today I have completely new flooring in my room that thankfully was covered by insurance. Gratitude leads to acceptance. Today I have a completely new career path that I am wildly excited about. Hopefully, there will a paycheck soon, but meanwhile, I have enough for today. Thank you for that. Gratitude leads to acceptance.

Call to Action:
Say thank-you to things that you don't think are supposed to be happening. See what happens.

# 270

## NEVER TOO LATE TO DEVELOP WILLINGNESS

*My friend Cordelia* said yesterday that she is now willing to make more self-loving food choices at age 79. Enough said.

Dear God,
Thank You for putting people like Cordelia in my life. Please remind me continually through the example of others that as long as I have a pulse, it is never too late to do anything!

Call to Action:
Think of something that you have been unwilling to do. Remember: it is never too late to develop willingness.

# 271

## ALLOWING MYSELF THE RIGHT TO "RUIN" OTHER PEOPLE'S DAY

*I remember in my late 20s* when I became free from other people's opinion of my body. Finally, I stopped letting other people's possible judgment dictate what clothes I wore. I put down the hammer and tore up "Sally's rules on how you need to look before you wear XYZ."

When I realized I had rights, I became liberated. Why isn't my body good enough to be uncovered like everyone else's?

Why can't I wear a sleeve-less top and a jean miniskirt? Why can't I wear silhouette-bearing clothing to the gym, or anywhere for that matter? Am I going to inconvenience someone or ruin his or her day?

Call to Action:
What item of clothing have you not been letting yourself wear because of your own personal rules on how your body needs to look before you wear it? Wear it because you have rights. Exercise your rights, even if it means risking ruining someone's day!

# 272

## SHOPPING FOR CLOTHES THAT ACTUALLY FIT NOW

*Over 30 years ago,* when I began my journey to live in a right-sized body no matter what was required, I was in my late 20s. At the time, I always wore sweats, except when I wore my flight attendant's uniform, which was too small for me, but I wore it anyway because I could not afford to replace it.

To my great surprise, the journey did not begin with weight loss. It began with radical acceptance of the body I was in at the time. It began with buying some clothes besides sweats that fit me. The reason for that was that my wise friend Cordelia suggested that before I could lose any weight, I would need to love my body exactly as is. I thought about that. It was hard for me to conceptualize something intangible like love of my body. What was a tangible thing that could symbolize love of my body?

That day, I made the best decision of my life. I tore up my "Rule Book" and embarked on an altogether new journey to health and healing. That day was such a pivotal day for me that I still remember exactly where I was … and I celebrate the day every year. It was the day I decided to allow myself to purchase clothing besides sweats: something that I liked, something in colors I liked, and something that fit my body on that day. Not something I intentionally purchased a little smaller than would fit because, don't you know, I am going to "diet" my way into fitting into it by some means of unhealthy and rigid food restriction. I bought two outfits. That was all I could afford. And I alternated them for months. That was the first day of my Big Amazing Life.

I am so grateful that I listened to that still, small voice on August 8, 1984.

Call to Action:

1. Honor your curves. Be willing to give yourself permission to wear silhouette-bearing clothes.

2. Ask a safe friend to accompany you clothes-shopping if you need help determining what clothes look like on you when they fit you.

# 273

## FALL IN LOVE WITH YOURSELF BY FILMING YOU

*Originally, when social media became a thing,* I turned up my nose at it with my usual contempt prior to investigation of anything new. Why do people need to communicate that way? Can't we just get together? Why do people have to post a public birthday greeting to their children? Can't they just tell them in person? But was that really the problem I had with social media—or was it something else?

Then COVID-19 came along. To make sense of the new normal that for me meant no source of income, I was forced to think outside the box and get a little creative. I thought about how I could do some sort of community service during a stressful time. The answer came to me: As a certified health coach, why not post quick tips to stay sane and boost your immune system? And so, it began. Other than that, I didn't put much thought into it. On the first video I shot, the words just came out of my mouth. As I write this, between March 22, 2020 and now, I have posted 99 times and counting. I have created content for everything from nutritious recipes to combating negative self-talk, to simple exercises to help with low back pain. I cannot believe I am saying this, but this has been quite a rewarding experience on many levels.

First, it has kept my morale up. With each successive posting, a new idea comes to me naturally and I cannot wait to video it. Second, it gives me a reason to dress in the morning. Third, it holds me accountable to the Universe, so if I have shared about daily Vitamin D walking, I'd better be doing it myself. Fourth, and most surprising, my body image has improved. I had already felt like my body image was good, but apparently there was room for improvement I hadn't known was possible at age 60! I have fallen in love with myself and my body on a deeper level. Sometimes I have posted with no makeup on. I lived through it. I've filmed in shorts with my wrinkled, pale legs and my wrinkled, yet somewhat muscular arms. The unexpected result is I am falling more deeply in love with myself. Sometimes as I edit a video of myself, I smile, seeing my late mother's mannerisms in me. If I hadn't been open-minded enough to venture out on this mission, I might never have experienced that deeper healing and pure joy.

Dear God,
Thank You for the gift of willingness to try new things at any age. It's never too late in life to wear shorts. I deserve to wear tank tops, no matter my size. It's never too late in life to heal from body dysmorphia on yet a deeper level.

Call to Action:
Fall in love with yourself by filming yourself and sharing with safe friends.

# 274
## OCULAR MIGRAINE

*Sadly, several of my friends* experience migraine headaches. Fortunately, I still have not had what I would call a meno-pause-related migraine. But recently I took an early morning bike ride, so early it was still dark outside. And suddenly I was experiencing spinning circles of light in both eyes.

Of course, I ignored it as I always tend to do with any unfamiliar ailment, hoping it would go away. It didn't. It kept happening. It got so bad that I had to end my bike ride sooner than planned. At breakfast, I googled my spinning circles of light issue and was freaked out to learn that "detached retina" was listed as one of the possible reasons for my eyes reacting as they did!

I was even more con-cerned when my optometrist scheduled an appointment

Dear God,
Thank You in advance for giving me the ability to stop pushing myself so hard. Retina gratitude, too.

for me that same day. Luckily, my retinas are intact, but I was told I'd experienced an ocular migraine and needed to stop pushing myself so hard.

# 275

## DEAR GOD, I FEEL ....

*Dear God,*
*I feel so tired. As usual, I've gotten myself into a situation*
*where I've got one too many things on my plate and I'm*
*exhausted. Unable to stop doing that. Will You help me?*
*Love, Sally*

*Dear Sally-Girl,*
*I think COVID-19 exhaustion is setting in for you, sweetie.*
*Can we make more realistic expectations about what you*
*can accomplish each day of*
*quarantine—or any day for*
*that matter? That sounds*
*like a good idea to Me.*
*That sounds right. And if*
*your goals are not met,*
*so be it. Trust Me.*
*Love, God*

Call to Action:
List two expectations you
have of yourself that are
unrealistic. Now explain
how each expectation could
be lowered a bit and thus
be accomplished.

# 276
## AWARDS AND THE POWER OF ACCOUNTABILITY

*I received a voice text* from my friend Cordelia today.

"OMG, I finally emailed Ted the investment guy from four years ago and I feel like I'm gonna throw up. I don't know why that is such a stressor, but I wrote the email, I sent the email and I asked for help, and there it is. Go me! Award!"

Sometimes things are scary for me to do. My response is to avoid them ... for weeks ... for months. Sometimes the months turn into years. I loved this message from Cordelia because it reminded me of how I took over ten years to complete a living trust. Hearing her imperfections and fears gives me permission to have imperfections and fears, too. I can let myself off the hook. It gives me permission to be imperfect. It causes me to look at what I am so afraid of.

When I break it down, mostly I am afraid that the person I need to speak with will discover I am not an expert in

XYZ. But it is kind of expected since that is why I am hiring the person. And if the person judges me or is condescending, I can certainly find another person in that field to help me.

Call to Action:
Is there a person you need to contact who you are giving too much power to?

# 277

## DESCARTES, INTENTIONAL IMPERFECTION & CHOICE

*Apparently,* the whole debate about perfectionism goes way back. Like, way back. René Descartes' work, *Meditations on the First Philosophy,* was originally written in Latin in 1641. He wrote:

"When I look more closely at myself and inquire into the nature of my errors, I notice that they depend on two concurrent cases, namely on the faculty of knowledge which is in me, and on the faculty of choice, or freedom of the will...I cannot produce any reason to prove that God ought to have given me a greater faculty of knowledge than He did...I [also] cannot complain that the will or freedom of choice which I received from God is not sufficiently extensive or perfect, since I know by experience that it is not restricted in any way. Indeed, I think it is very noteworthy that there is nothing else in me which is so perfect and so great."

Why do I make mistakes?

René Descartes, a brilliant mathematician and philosopher who lived in France, believed that we can make mistakes because God intentionally gave us freedom of will. Descartes argues that there is nothing more desirable than this freedom.

So, in seeking perfection, am I defying what God intended for me? His words make me go, "Hmm."

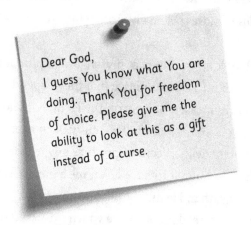

Dear God,
I guess You know what You are doing. Thank You for freedom of choice. Please give me the ability to look at this as a gift instead of a curse.

# 278

## FIXING VS. HOLDING A SPACE FOR YOUR FEELINGS

*I was on the phone* with my friend Cordelia (73) yesterday. She mentioned she had an appointment with a cardiologist later that day. And that her back hurt. She thought maybe she needed back surgery for a condition she has called stenosis. Immediately, the health coach and the "other-oriented fixer" in me kicked in and several suggestions lined up in my vocal region, quite eager to come out of my mouth. AND, I must admit, there was some judgment on my part. She has asked for nutrition suggestions from me in the past, but has never followed any of them. Still, I love her. I paused, took a breath, and held back my comments.

As she continued, I didn't speak other than to make sounds to acknowledge I heard her. I realized all that she wanted was for me to listen, not to fix. She was processing her thoughts and feelings, weighing her options. All that was expected of me was to hold a space for her feelings. Amazingly, I did just that. Huge progress for me.

Dear God,
Thank You for giving me the ability to listen today. Help me to remember three things before speaking: Is it kind? Is it true? Is it necessary?

# 279

## THE SHELTER-IN-PLACE EXPERIENCE

*I have heard countless stories* about people's shelter-in-place experiences with COVID-19. There are as many different situations and solutions as there are people in the world. I honor and send sincere gratitude for all the people on the front line. Some people are virtually paralyzed, emotionally eating and honoring that. For whatever reason, their response is cocooning or hibernating to store energy for when the time comes. I honor these people. Others are taking stock of their lives and careers to dramatically pivot both in a major way. I honor these people as well.

I can't help wondering if people will experience a similar struggle once we reenter our old routines, post-COVID-19. And if that's the case, what can we learn from this experience?

My biggest takeaway is a renewed acceptance of where each person is in their life. This is a brilliant reminder that judgment is a waste of time. If I liken the COVID-19 pandemic to aging in general, isn't honoring each person where she is a great perspective to take? And therefore, how can we help and support each other to thrive?

The shelter-in-place experience in me honors the shelter-in-place experience in you.

The aging experience in me honors the aging experience in you.

Dear God,
Please give me the ability not to judge others today. Help me remember the less I judge others the less I judge myself.

# 280

## No Siren = No Emergency

*Even after 30 years of living a Big Amazing Life,* my beautiful, creative, addictive personality tries to take me down. It can be incredibly resourceful and creative. Lately I've noticed it likes to tell me I am behind … on everything. Everything is an emergency and I need to respond immediately. 911. Obviously responding to multiple tasks is impossible, so you can see how crazymaking this thought process is. This self-imposed state of emergency is yet another way I try to control outcomes. I try to exert my will instead of surrendering to the will of a Power greater than myself. Basically, if left to my own devices, I am the

Dear God,
Please give me the ability to discern the difference between realistic expectations and emergencies. Give me the willingness to give You the wheel. I will be here in the back seat.

poster child for Self-Will Run Riot. To make matters worse, as I age, this MO could lead to a heart attack as it did in my own father twice.

The solution is another mnemonic. When I am self-imposing emergencies in my day, I can call an accountability partner and hear myself say aloud, "I don't hear a siren, so this is not an emergency."

# 281

## Don't Believe the Lies

*Lately I've been telling myself* that I am not a good mom because I am not available for my college-aged son the way I should be.

"You are a failure. You are not present. You are modeling how he will treat his future wife. How dare you not drop everything and do his laundry and spend every waking moment with him."

He just knocked on the door to my office. I put aside my computer and we talked for a few minutes. We discussed our plans for the day. He handed me a card. In it he had written:

> *I am so lucky to have such a phenomenal mother who continues to chase her dreams and adapt to the constantly changing world of today. I aspire to be like you.*

Call to Action: What lies are you believing today?

Like I said, don't believe the lies.

# 282

## PUT IT ON PAPER

*In my twenties* I began a journey to recover from disordered eating and disordered body image. Journal-writing was recommended by professionals and others I worked with. I judged the suggestion. How stupid. That's something young girls do. How can that be valuable? What if someone reads it? What if someone reads my innermost thoughts and feelings and laughs at me? Sees my dark side? What if someone I'm writing about reads what I've written? It's just too vulnerable.

Yet I had to admit, the people who suggested I write had qualities I wanted. I guess I could find a place where my writing would be safe. It got to the point where I was so unhappy in my life that my emotional pain was greater than the discomfort of risking someone reading my journal. I finally was willing to give it a try, against my better judgment. This is how my brain worked: I would try writing, it wouldn't work, and I would happily report the failure to the people who suggested it and return to my small miserable life.

# 283
## WRITING AND BEING VULNERABLE

*I write a lot.* I freely share writing techniques I love with others who are in pain, in the hope that it will bring them relief and inspire their healing journey. Writing is healing. I love writing because it results in my feeling better.

Surprisingly, not everyone who wants to feel better is willing to write. I thought it was a stupid waste of time when it was first suggested to me. I had my usual response of contempt prior to investigation. I have come to realize that I initially scoffed because I didn't want to be vulnerable. Writing can involve being vulnerable, especially writing to a power greater than myself.

Call to Action:
Be willing to try writing and risk being vulnerable. Commit to write one sentence with the option to write more. What have you got to lose but your isolation and discomfort?

For me, I've come to realize writing is a no-brainer because I want to live my best life. Writing has brought me relief and healing on multiple levels. Most importantly, writing enables me to be vulnerable. It takes courage to be vulnerable. Vulnerability increases connection. I want to connect. Connection is like my medicine. I must be vulnerable to have faith.

# 284
## TURNING WANTS INTO INTENTIONS INTO GOALS INTO REALITY

*By this point in your life,* you've probably heard or read numerous things about goal setting. Before you yawn and get distracted, maybe thinking about what you'll have for lunch today, hear me out. Last week I heard yet another talk on goal setting and I was able to hear it on a much deeper level than ever before—physically, intellectually, emotionally, and spiritually. Whether it's about personal growth, career pivot, money, or all three, there is something powerful about setting a specific, measurable goal with a timeline.

Recently a large coaching group for women I'm a member of was given a goal challenge to find an extra $100 in one week that we were not planning on. I had objections. "How stupid" is usually my first response to anything. "What good will $100 do? It won't even make a dent in my debt. Besides, I'm too busy."

But I respect the leader of the group, so I allowed the idea to take up some space in my head, which was a big deal for me. I had no sooner allowed this idea into my head before even more objections arose. "The women in this group are not where I am. Either they are way more evolved in their businesses than I or they probably aren't required to succeed in business because they have a spouse's income to fall back on if things don't work out." It was my usual black and white thinking. My usual "terminal uniqueness" appeared. I'm either less than or better than. Terminal uniqueness is one of the ways I avoid connecting with my fellow humans to avoid feelings and vulnerability.

Realizing this, I took contrary action and remained open to the idea. I wrote down $100 on a Post-it. The leader went on to give the "proper goal-setting" talk and used the example of this $100 challenge outlining the three components:

Specific: Find an extra $100 you weren't planning on
Measurable: $100
Time Limit: 1 week

I went on with my day. The next day someone unexpectedly gave me $60. What? Could this be …? By the end of the week, I found $40 in a desk drawer. What? Always the skeptic, I dismissed the possibility that this had anything to do with that goal.

A week later, there was another coaching session. The leader exuberantly recounted all the stories she'd received from roughly 100 women. The total amount of money people reported was in the tens of thousands. I had met my $100 goal with extraordinarily little thought or effort. I hadn't even reported my result to the group. I connected the dots. I got it: if the simple act of writing $100 on a Post-it resulted in $100, how much more could I accomplish if I put more intention into where I want to go in my life?

Dear Universe,
Remind me that the definition of insanity is repeating the same behavior and expecting a different result. Open my mind to putting my ideas and intentions on paper so that I may break through long-standing barriers to being the person I know in my heart I am meant to be.

Call to Action:
I know it's scary. But be willing to go there and trust yourself.

Do you want something? Are you ready to stop self-sabotaging and make progress? Why not turn it into a goal? Goals are powerful because you can measure them to know if you are on track. Even if it's uncomfortable and scary, you know exactly what the finish line is. It's the goal (objective) you set for yourself.

# 285

## TRY SOMETHING NEW AGAINST YOUR "BETTER JUDGMENT"

They say necessity is the mother of invention. My income virtually evaporated overnight when COVID-19 required global social distancing. Paralyzed with fear of failure, I contemplated teaching a movement class on Zoom. No way! I cannot possibly do that. My mentors can do it, but I have nowhere near the skills and presenting experience they do. Literally hundreds of excuses filled my head. Then other instructors posted on social media: "It's okay if you don't choose to pivot to online." Phew. Still, there was the issue of no income and a mortgage to pay. It was imperative that I reconsider walking through this fear.

I watched three of my fitness instructor mentors present on Zoom. I took copious notes. I could do that. I got up the courage to put my own choreography together. But I wasn't confident enough to market myself. A friend offered to help me market. That felt extremely uncomfortable, yet I was willing to sit with the feelings without quitting. The big day drew near. I practice-taught friends through Zoom. I taught a one-on-one session to one of my private clients. My Zoom connection repeatedly froze up. The client was extremely frustrated and elected not to continue until she could come in person again. I accepted this as a sign it wasn't meant to be.

Upon further analysis, I realized it wasn't the technological aspect of using virtual communication that bothered me, it was the inevitability of teaching to people who I had never met, whose bodies I was unfamiliar with. How could I cue them at the level I preferred? My learned coping mechanisms of perfectionism, people-pleasing, and temperature-taking clouded my judgment. And how could I teach to people who didn't already know me and love me? I'd always relied on getting in-person, immediate feedback cues from people I worked with. With this technology, these cues would be nearly impossible to pick up through my smart phone, with multiple people simultaneously. I almost let the fear and discomfort stop me … almost. But I didn't.

Something inside me pulled me forward. Now is the time. Just do it. Let go of perfection. Let go of people's opinion, of you. Open your heart to helping people. You've got this. Today I teach my fifth class online and have plans to teach a new series. It would have been simply fine if I opted not to walk through this fear. Something inside said, "Just do this one time." I listened. I'm so glad I did.

Dear God,
Thank You for the courage to walk through being new at something. Please keep reminding me that's what life is about. Gently remind me about this when I go back to thinking it's all about looking good.

Call to Action:
What is your one thing? Now is the time. Just do it. Let go of perfection. Let go of people's opinions of you. Open your heart to helping people. You've got this.

# 286

## UNORTHODOX PRAYER IS STILL PRAYER

*Influenced by my formal religious upbringing,* I always felt as if my prayers had to be composed with an eloquent style, the way our minister's were. His booming voice was always comforting, and I loved when his huge warm hand shook mine as we exited the sanctuary. I know they told us to pray in between Sunday sermons, but I mistakenly thought that my prayers needed to be as carefully worded as our minister's. Thinking that was impossible, I used that reasoning as an excuse and therefore rarely prayed. Sadly, I was the one who suffered from this shortsightedness.

In my mid-twenties, I was taught simply that prayer is talking to God and meditation is listening to God … period. This information gave me permission to find a concept of God I could do business with. It gave me the freedom to connect with God in my own language. It reminded me that God wanted to get to know me as me. If He wasn't strong enough to handle all my feelings, I needed to find a new concept of my God. What a revelation.

For me, the content of the prayer is not the point as much as the actual effort to connect with a Power Greater than myself. Some days, my prayer is simple and direct.

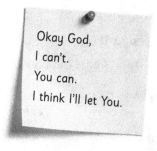

Okay God,
I can't.
You can.
I think I'll let You.

# 287

## SOCIAL MEDIA PREOCCUPATION

*This morning* I am preoccupied with turning off all the little red circular notification lights on my social-media app icons on my phone. It is driving me crazy because there's one I simply cannot figure out how to turn off. I have clicked every possible place. I am a little embarrassed to give it enough power to write about it. But I do so to illustrate a point.

> Dear God,
> Please give me the ability to let go of distractions that keep me from connecting with my fellow humans and from connecting with You.

Underlying this mindset and behavior is most likely a feeling I am avoiding. What is it? I go outside and stand quietly as I watch the leaves on my poplar tree move with the gentle morning breeze. I am transported. The feelings come. I am presenting a live event later today where

I will interview a guest. I'm nervous. Will I come off as polished as some of my mentors do? I realize maybe it doesn't matter. What matters most is that I focus on and connect with my guest and be myself. That's a great person to be.

Call to Action:
Is there something you're fixated on today? Are you willing to look beneath to determine if it's not about the red circular notification lights on your social media?

# 288

## NOT BEING AN EXPERT

*I love being an expert.* I love telling you I have already mastered "such and such" and telling you how you can, too. I was working on a project where learning a new job skill was required, and I was uncomfortable ... extremely. My stomach was in knots over learning a new skill. I thought I was incapable of learning to create the educational video I needed to create for work. The process lasted for over a month. It required endless patience and faith in myself. It required acting as if I had confidence in myself. It would have been much easier to go back to my familiar, comfortable day job. I really wanted to do that. It would have been much easier to eat junk food with wild abandon to avoid my uncomfortable feelings. I did that for a day, but I decided it wasn't working. In the end, I stuck with it. I am so glad I did. The video is awesome.

I'm not an expert videographer and I may never "master" producing educational videos. But I can tell you to believe in yourself. I can tell you to keep practicing. I can encourage you to keep giving yourself permission not to be an expert at the new thing. I can suggest that you be patient with yourself and lower your expectations about how long something will take to get the hang of. I can tell you to let yourself feel super icky and uncomfortable, yet NOT quit. Repeatedly I can tell myself these things as well. Together we can do this.

Call to Action:
Be willing to sit with the discomfort and learn a new skill.

Dear God,
Please give me the courage and patience required today to sit through uncomfortable feelings and help me remember that learning new skills is so worth it. Please remind me that putting pressure on myself to be an expert in all things is too heavy a burden.

# 289

## FAITH CONQUERS SHAME

*I was expected to learn a new skill recently.* My business partner suggested a new project for me. I hate not being an expert. I had no idea how to do it. How would I if I had never done it before? Why was it so hard to give myself grace? If my son were doing something for the first time, I would give him grace. If you were doing something for your first time, I would give you grace. I realized that shame was rearing its head. I would need extreme faith to conquer my shame.

Faith is a key ingredient for me in overcoming shame each time I experience it. My business partner suggested I go live on social media and tell my eating disorder story. Not just my usual light-hearted, silly, 1-minute impromptu-type video that I create almost daily with little thought. That video takes under 30 minutes to create, edit, and post. She meant a 10-15 minute live presentation where I was completely vulnerable. I have never done such a thing. Just hearing the suggestion made my stomach hurt.

When she first suggested I do this, I ignored her for about a week, hoping she would forget about it. She didn't. Next, she gave me a loose framework for the presentation, outlining what information she wanted it to contain. Not being experienced in extemporaneous speaking, it became evident that a script would be required for part of this. The project gave me a stomachache each time I contemplated it. Yet, against my better judgment, I called on my faith and chose to tackle it. I developed the outline into a script and returned it to her.

Each time she read my latest draft; she would politely return it to me with suggestions about how to make it better. This went back and forth many times. For a recovering perfectionist like me, naturally I took it personally each time she told me it wasn't quite right yet. She is less than half my age so WTF! Inside, I laughed at myself, admitting she knew way more than I did. Each time I felt uncomfortable, wanted to quit, exercised my faith, and did it anyway, despite loud protests from my head. I welcomed the opportunity to work on humility.

I tend to be capable in a lot of areas in life, so it was quite frustrating when it became apparent that this was not going to be a "one-and-done" filming experience. I rehearsed. It was nowhere near the quality we wanted. Deflated, I wanted to quit again. If doing this was part of being an entrepreneur, maybe I'd rather go back to my day job. I spontaneously ate cookies and vanilla bean ice cream that night. Before quitting, I decided to go to bed and sleep on it. Maybe things would look different in the morning. They did.

We edited the script some more and I rehearsed again. It was better, but still nowhere near what we were hoping for. The arduous process took several more edits and practice sessions before we were both happy with the result.

One more time, I was reminded that sometimes extreme faith and patience are called for. But the result makes it all worth it.

**S** hould

**H** ave

**A** lready

**M** astered

**E** verything

**NOPE.**

*Dear Big Love,*
*Thank You in advance for giving me the ability to show myself the same grace You show me when I attempt something for the first time.*

*Dear Sally-Girl,*
*I am so completely blown away by your courage and willingness to try new things lately! I am so proud of you! Way to go! Award!*
*Love, Big Love*

# 290

## EXTERNAL VALIDATION AND REFILLING THE BIRD FEEDER

*I wake up.* I'm not that excited about today. There's no external validation (EV) coming my way that I can think of. There is nothing wrong with receiving external validation, but when I need it to face the day … that can be problematic.

Therefore, when I wake up expecting EV, it's a sign I need to believe in myself more: to look within; to look to my God; to connect with myself and my God. What physical action can I take to reconnect spiritually? I notice my bird-feeder is empty. Bird feeders are not allowed in my condo complex, so it's hidden inconspicuously within a bush in my front yard. That way, it isn't seen when conduct inspections are randomly made in my neighborhood. Because it's against the rules, it's a hassle to refill because some of my neighbors (one in particular) might report me.

I decide it's early enough that most of my neighbors aren't up and around yet. I sneak out and recover the feeder and refill it in my garage. It's successfully rehung within a matter of minutes. I'm not sure whether it's the knowing anticipation of bird songs outside my window or the fact that I have pulled off a stealth mission, but I am filled with a renewed sense of purpose. It's probably a little of both. One more time, I am dumbfounded at how little effort it takes to shift from KF*** to KJOY euphoria. Willingness and action are the magic words.

Dear God,
Thank You for bird songs that make my heart sing, too.

Call to Action:
Find your validation today.

# 291

## TEN CHAIR STANDS

*It might sound silly* but even as a fitness and wellness coach for over 20 years, some days I cannot decide what to do for exercise. Or I have trouble prioritizing my day. There are several things I want to accomplish, but instead I sit paralyzed, with my head swirling.

Days like this are ten chair stand days. It works my glutes, my abs, and my thighs. It elevates my heart rate a little. It produces endorphins. It helps clarify my priorities and gets me moving forward with the business of living.

Dear God,
Please give me knowledge of Your will for me today and the power to carry that out.

Call to Action:
Try ten chair stands and see what happens.

# 292

## COMPULSIVE DOING ACCOUNTABILITY

*I consider myself a recovering Human-Doing.* From the moment I awake each day, I am unconsciously pushing myself to do more. A cousin of workaholism, "compulsive doing," as it is also referred to, is another another way my addictive personality manifests itself. I sometimes erroneously brag about this trait or feel "better than" those not afflicted with it when, in fact, it is nothing to brag about. Like all addictive personality traits, nothing is ever enough, so whatever I accomplish in each day falls short and self-criticism ensues. On top of that, it keeps me from connecting with my fellow humans.

Like many Human-Doers, I tend to be way too hard on myself. There are times at the end of the day when I critique myself, falling short of some insanely high expectation. When that happens, I call my friend Cordelia (43) who shares this character trait. We both want to overcome this intimacy barrier. Our shared weakness connects us to each other, enabling a more powerful healing.

We use an accountability tool we have developed to help us right-size our Human-Doing tendencies. It works equally well, no matter which one of us is suffering. For example, the other day I called her and relayed the ginormous list of things I had done that day, asking for an award. She enthusiastically proclaimed into the phone, "Freaking AWARD, lady!" After the call, she followed up with an emoji of a trophy and clapping hands.

When I heard myself recount aloud the list of "all I got done for the day," it even surprised me because I had completely forgotten how much I'd done. We laughed our heads off about how cute we are, and the self-beating fell away.

Of course, being efficient can be a good thing. I am incredibly efficient, and I can get a crap-ton done in a day. But it can also be a dangerous thing when I fail to stop and appreciate the moment. And I miss out on opportunities to connect with people I love. As is always the case, balance is queen.

Dear God,
Help me remember to keep my eyes open today so I can see what You have in store for me.

# 293

## BRUSH YOUR TEETH WITH YOUR EYES CLOSED

*One of the tools I use* to slow myself down is to brush my teeth with my eyes closed. It might sound silly, but this forces me literally to focus where my feet are. As I stand there brushing, I first bring my awareness to my feet. Next, I notice whether I have equal weight distribution on each foot. Then I notice if my weight is balanced between the balls of my feet and my heels. It brings me back to being a human being.

Dear God,
Please slow me down today. Give me the ability not to rush myself.

Call to Action:
Make a point of spending time in the present today. What can you do to spend one minute where your feet are?

# 294
## GRATEFUL FOR MY DOCTOR

*My friend Cordelia* (40) lamented to me that she had been gaining weight in her mid-section over the past several months. She had spoken with her gynecologist and asked if it could be due to shifting hormones as she approached menopause. Her doctor told her that because she is still getting her period it could not possibly be hormone-related. She then told Cordelia she should just work out more and eat fewer carbs.

Clearly this doctor does not know my friend because if she had any idea of the type, duration, and frequency of her work outs, she would never have said that. In my head, I thought, "Time for a new doctor." Thankfully, Cordelia said the very same words aloud.

Reflection:
How fortunate I am that my gynecologist treats my symptoms rather than making broad generalizations.

# 295

## PERIMENOPAUSAL SHIFTS: OILY HAIR & SKIN

*One day my friend Cordelia* complained to me about how perimenopausal shifts affected her hair. Her once-beautiful curly hair had become so oily that she now had to lather and rinse at least twice each time she washed it. All her life, her hair had been so dry that she wouldn't even use shampoo, just conditioner.

"And then there's my skin," she continued. She said it hadn't been this oily since puberty. I listened, making under-standing sounds as she continued. Sometimes you just need a place to get it all out. When

Dear God,
Help me to be a compassionate listener. Help me to be of service when the opportunity arises. Getting out of my head is a good thing and this friendship is important to me.

she seemed to have finished, I commiserated and added that I had never expected to have acne after 20. We laughed about how our bodies are changing and throwing us unexpected curveballs.

# 296

## Body Dysmorphia Reset & Healing

*Even in my late 20s,* after my body had returned to a moderate adult-sized body, I disliked having my photo taken. I believe the issue stemmed from my overweight days coupled with lingering body dysmorphia. In childhood, my well-meaning mother would often give me tips on what to wear to look thinner, how to stand, and how to sit to look best. I took it a little too much to heart. I misunderstood her message to be: *If you don't always look your best, you will be unlovable, alone, and lonely forever.*

When I would see the picture after it was taken, it activated severe self-criticism. There was also self-comparison if someone was in the photo with me. I always fell short. I was hyper-critical of myself. The negative self-talk that ensued was unpleasant to say the least. It just got to the point where I avoided being in pictures and avoided looking at pictures of myself because it wasn't worth the mental self-abuse. What's with the whole selfie revolution? It's a hard NO from me.

A few years back, my friend Cordelia showed me a perfectly fine photo of herself that her husband had taken of her while she was walking. She was wearing jeans, boots, and a leather jacket. The only skin showing was her face, but she complained about how unattractive she felt. She cited her sagging skin and butt and her wrinkles, etc. In my opinion, she looked like the adorable friend I know and love. It was evident that the picture made her cringe. She could barely bring herself to show it to me, yet I could find absolutely nothing negative about it.

"Does feeling unattractive ever go away?" she asked.

Then it occurred to me. She was experiencing body dysmorphia. Seeing it so clearly in another caused a powerful moment of clarity for me. It instantaneously catapulted my body-dysmorphia healing to a new level. I am not saying it's completely removed, but that day something in me shifted and I have experienced a newfound willingness to self-love ever since, at a deeper level than I had known before.

Dear God,
Please help me continue to heal from crippling body dysmorphia. It prevents me from connecting on a deeper level with my fellow humans. It blocks me from the sunlight of the Spirit.

Call to Action:
Has body dysmorphia outlived its usefulness in your life? Are you willing to look deeper?

# 297

## OUTDATED BREATHING, POSTURE, & CORE MINDSETS

*Recently I met with my friend Cordelia (46).* She attends a mat Pilates class I teach. It is possible she is living by outdated breathing, posture, and core mindsets. I surmise this because she asked me why I don't make the class "harder." I get this question all the time when women haven't yet embraced the importance of developing core awareness and maintaining core strength. I used to fall into that category myself.

When I was her age, I didn't much care about core awareness, either. My reasoning was, "why would I spend time focusing on my breathing, posture, and core when I could get the immediate feedback of an endorphin buzz by recruiting my large, global mobilizer muscles doing a bunch of lunges, planks, and squats? Why would I care about the firing order of muscles at multiple levels all the way down to the minute local stabilizer level? Why would

I care if I consciously considered skeletal positioning while doing the moves? That took too much thought. I just wanted to zone out while exercising. I only have so much time in my busy day." What I hadn't realized at the time was that I was basing my thinking on the body I had at age 20.

I was living by outdated breathing, posture, and core mindsets. At 20, I was healthy, pain-free, and flexible. Awareness of breathing, posture, and core had an incredibly low priority. Basically, I could do any athletic task I set out to do, with little to no forethought or warm-up. In my 30s, I once did a mini-triathlon without any preparation. Even at age 39, I rode my bike in the Solvang Century (100 hilly miles) with about four weeks of pretraining. The longest distance I'd ridden prior to that was 30 miles on one ride.

Little did I know or care about the massive role hormone levels played in keeping my body in this highly functioning state. I didn't need to spend a lot of time thinking about my breathing, posture, and core because gravity hadn't caught up with me. My hormone levels were optimal, and my body was a "finely tuned machine."

But in my 40s when those hormone levels began shifting, I realized breathing, posture, and core needed to have a much higher priority. My perspective from my 20s had outlived its usefulness. I wasn't living in a 20-year-old body anymore, and engaging my core needed to become a higher priority to optimize the physiology of this older body at the cellular level. The upright posture and skeletal positioning that I once had taken for granted had now become something I needed to approach with intention to sustain it.

If this sounds extreme, contemplate the next round-backed, forward-headed older woman you see in the grocery store. Why has she chosen a full-sized grocery cart, when she is only purchasing one or two items? It's because she needs to hold onto the cart for support to get through the store without falling. She has lost touch with her center of gravity. She has continued to live in the posture mindset from her 20-year-old body where it was less important to focus on her breathing, posture, and core, but that mindset has long outlived its usefulness. There definitely needs to be a place for breath, core awareness, and strengthening in my workouts today if I don't want to be that old woman in the grocery store. My mantra: ears over shoulders over hips over ankles over feet.

Dear God,
Please continue to remind me to give breathing, posture, and core awareness an age- and hormone level-appropriate priority today.

Call to Action:
Look at your breathing, posture, and core mindset. Is it age- and hormone-level appropriate? And don't worry. You can still enjoy that endorphin buzz that comes from recruiting larger muscle groups. Just make sure the small, core muscles are recruited first. Win-Win!

# 298
## Labial Fusion

I met my friend Cordelia (46) for coffee today and we had our usual lively conversation that jumped from lip gloss to vibrators and everything in between. There's never an agenda with us, and frequent subject pivots are almost a requirement. I find this type of non sequitur banter quite refreshing. It makes my heart feel carefree, as I am forced to stop taking myself too seriously as we giggle at the ridiculous.

Suddenly she leaned in, her body language and half whisper signaling a shift to a more intimate topic.

"Oh, did I tell you about my last visit to my OB/Gyn? I have labial fusion." Some people have the type of fusion where the two sides partially join. Hers is the type where her labia fuse

Dear God,
Thank You for my women friends who are comfortable sharing their very personal female issues with me. It is so comforting to know that I am trusted with confidential information.

apart, away from each other, instead of the type where they fuse toward each other. Apparently, this is a condition that can arise when estrogen levels decrease.

# 299

## DECLUTTER KITCHEN COUNTER

*The voices in my head can be quite cruel.* If I believe them and dwell on them, the result is almost certain stagnation. The good news is, they are easily distracted. Usually even the smallest positive action can get me off the Doomsday Train and headed in a new, better direction.

Today the voices in my head loom large. They are saying I don't know what I am doing … that I'm a failure. The uncertainty of life plagues me today … that I will never amount to anything. My full potential will never be realized because fear will always dominate me and paralyze me. Wow, and it's not even 8:00 a.m. yet.

Today is a good day for a ten-minute declutter challenge. Set the timer

Dear God,
Please give me the faith to face the unknown today despite my fears. Help me override negative voices in my head.

for ten minutes. Then pick one small, cluttered area of the house, such as the kitchen counter. Put things in their proper places until the timer beeps. Something about giving my brain a concrete task distracts it from berating me.

Call to Action:
Take the 10-Minute Declutter Challenge. Now move to another room with the timer and give the challenge another go!

# 300
## YOUR FOOD IS FINE

*Discussion about food and weight is common.* I hear it all the time, not just because I work in fitness and wellness coaching.

"I can't believe how much I have been eating lately."

"I'm trying to be good."

"I'm on the XYZ diet."

In over 30 years of maintaining a 35-lb. weight loss without dieting or employing what I call "diet mentality," I have watched a lot of fad diets come and go. Dieting not only perpetuated my problem, but it also kept me from looking within to discover my healthy, normal, and appropriate feelings.

Dear God,
Thank You for giving me the strength and the vision to stop dieting and get out of diet mentality all those years ago. I am so grateful not to be in that club anymore. Help me remember that, no matter how uncomfortable and unfamiliar, feeling my feelings will not kill me.

The same goes for being critical of my food choices at any given meal. Beating myself up for my less-than-perfect food choices also separates me from the present, from my fellow humans, and from my feelings. It doesn't serve me in any way. It blocks me from healing on any level.

Call to Action:
What if your weight is just where it is supposed to be today? What would you be free to feel?

# 301
## ASK FOR GUIDANCE & CHANGE THE LIGHT BULB

As with most days, I begin by reviewing my mental to-do list. Once again, today's list consists of enough tasks for about seven days, rather than just this one. And they all are equally high priorities in my compulsive-doer brain. There are the two significant work projects. Showering: Wash hair or not? Hair washing takes longer. Grocery shopping? Thank heavens I have already exercised, walked the dog, and eaten breakfast, or it would be even more of a conundrum.

Aware of my unrealistic expectations, I become frustrated, not knowing how to prioritize. I become anxious, cognizant of my tendency to be self-critical for not accomplishing enough. I future-trip the end of the day where I am beating myself up for not having done enough, and the only way to stop the self-beating is to eat spontaneously, which in turn leads to more self-criticism. It is only 7:15 a.m. and I am already fatigued by these mental gyrations. I catch myself. I smile and silently laugh at how adorable I am. I sit down, close my eyes, and ask the Universe how it wants to use me in a powerful way today.

I decide to replace that burned-out light bulb in my bathroom. I'm surprised at the heightened feeling of well-being that such a small act brings. I breathe deeply. I think I'll take a shower next and see how the day unfolds.

Dear God,

Use me in a powerful way today. Enable me to accept the things I accomplish today as exactly the right number. Give me the grace to choose self-loving foods and portion sizes today, amidst the distractions of my head and the world around me. Thank You in advance.

# 302

## STAYING CURRENT WITH FEELINGS/ AVOIDING SPONTANEOUS EATING

All I can think of is eating right now. There's no particular food on my mind. I just don't want to feel the way I feel right now, so I am obsessing on what I could eat to stop these feelings. When I experience this craving, writing helps me get in touch with these feelings.

> *Dear God,*
> *I feel uncomfortable because there is conflict in some of my relationships. I am reassessing my relationships and I'm realizing that some of them don't serve me anymore. Or even worse, some never served me at all. They never felt nurturing for me. I felt unsafe sharing my feelings for fear of being ridiculed. It wasn't like a blatant ridiculing. It was more like a subtle judging (as if that's not as bad?). In some relationships, when I parted company with the people, I felt drained rather than refreshed and joyful.*

*My part is that I have let these relationships go on for years because it was too uncomfortable to excuse myself from them.*
*Love, Sally*

*Dear Sally-Girl,*
*I know this is big for you. I know you're super uncomfortable. I support you in keeping only those relationships where you feel nurtured and safe. You don't need to be embarrassed. Please forgive yourself for staying in these types of relationships for so long, even if they have lasted years. I still love you. I always love you. I will help you let these relationships go with love. I will help you bless these people and wish them new loving relationships with others in the Universe. I will hold you in My arms while you walk through these uncomfortable self-care actions.*
*Love, God*

# 303
## Walking With Intention and Attention: Mind-Body Walking Revisited

Before my hormonal transition, I simply loved to walk. I would walk for hours and never feel the least bit fatigued. Walking was an activity that required no thought about anything. I could walk with a friend and talk simultaneously. Walking brought me so much joy, both physically and spiritually. The cardiovascular benefit combined with being in nature and fellowshipping with a fellow human. Win. Win. Win.

With the advent of my hormonal depletion, joint pain made walking less pleasant. If I'd been sitting for a while, such as at a meal or enjoying an iced tea with a friend, I would usually limp upon rising and walking away from the table. Often when I walked with a friend, keeping pace with her was arduous, painful, and stressful.

I experienced a deep sadness around this observation. Never being one to give up, I continued walking, despite the pain. I don't know what I expected, but there was just no way I was willing to give up this activity that I loved so much.

One day I stumbled on new information. I held my abdominals in. I really paid attention to my posture. I paid attention to my breath. I borrowed from the principles of posture and breathing that I use in Pilates. The pain decreased dramatically. It wasn't instantaneous, but I learned that if I walked with intention for about one-fourth mile or so, the pain dramatically decreased and so did my limp.

I created a whole process and I named it, of course, because I love giving everything a name. I call it Mind-Body Walking and it has four steps that were listed earlier in this book, but I've repeated them again for you:

1. Breathe in through the nose, out through the mouth with pursed lips.

2. Lift and separate your pec muscles.

3. Imagine a grape in your navel and squeeze the grape.

4. Supermodel walk. Swivel your hips a little. Walk like you are all that. Because you ARE.

Try different combinations of the ratio between length of breaths and steps such as: Breathe in for 4 steps, gently hold that inhale for 4 more steps; then exhale for 6 steps.

How much do I hate that I must pay such close attention to how I walk? … a ton. I never used to have to do that. How much do I miss mindless walking? … plenty. But I am grateful I can walk again, super grateful.

Dear God,
I feel sad because my parameters around walking have totally changed. Thank You for the ability to walk. Please help me with my attitude about what is.

# 304
## GRATITUDE

Dear God,

Here's what I am grateful for today:

Grateful my upper back hurts from sitting and not being willing to practice proper posture.

Grateful the awesome skin oil I use on my décolleté is causing acne.

Grateful my dog doesn't embrace visitors to our house.

Grateful my hair is frizzing today.

Grateful I am painfully aware I need to set an uncomfortable boundary with a friend.

Grateful my business is growing more slowly than I expect.

Grateful the source of my next paycheck is unknown.

Grateful I have hair.

Grateful I have all four limbs.

Grateful I have birds singing outside my window.

Grateful I have had the privilege of raising a son.

# 305
## Embrace the No for Today

*I am preparing my breakfast* and juicing my celery-grape-fruit combination supply for the next few days. I tend to get on a kick and stay with it until I'm sick of it. My fresh juiced celery-grapefruit combination coupled with an individual serving bag of lightly salted cashews has been my kick for about a year now and I still love them. Yes, an entire year. Bless my routine-loving soul.

I'm listening to a podcast my friend Cordelia (50) sent me, so my brain can focus. As I'm listening, I've got Cordelia on my mind. Meanwhile, it's been about two weeks now that I've been working on that project for work that requires me to learn a new skill. In the spirit of my usual unrealistic expectations, I am incredulous (while grinning at my cuteness) at the fact that the new skill is still not all polished. This means that the project is not yet finished.

A few days ago, my partner at work suggested I ask a friend to review my project. As usual when I receive a suggestion from someone, I said aloud, "Okay, that's an idea." I said silently, "No f-ing way! And besides, which one of my friends would be the right person to ask? I don't really trust my picker lately." Something I have learned about myself is that I am only as brave as I am on any given day. I honor and embrace that fact. I let it be okay that for today, I am not brave enough to ask someone to review my project.

*Dear Big Love,*
*I am too scared to even consider letting a friend review my project. And I can't even think which friend I would choose. This is hard.*
*Love, Sally*

*Dear Sally-Girl,*
*That is totally fine. I love you no matter what you decide. You are doing your absolute best. I love you no matter what you eat. I love you no matter what you weigh.*
*Love, Big Love*

# 306
## CRYING IS HEALING

*I continued creating drafts* for my work project for weeks. I continued to let it be okay that I was unwilling to ask a friend to review the project and give feedback. Then this morning I had a conversation with Big Love.

Big Love: You know that might be a good idea to have a friend review your project, Sally-Girl.

Me: Yeah, but that would mean asking for feedback and I can't take it.

Big Love: Why?

Me: Because I know my tendency to have unrealistic expectations. My unrealistic expectation is that she would say, "THAT IS THE BEST, MOST PERFECT THING I'VE EVER SEEN. ABSOLUTELY NO REVISIONS NEEDED!" Any feedback besides that would be unbearable for me.

Big Love: Why?

Me: Because I feel uncomfortable being that vulnerable with another person. This project is about my biggest passion in life. What if she laughs? What if there's the slightest awkward pause before she begins to give feedback, or just the slightest weird, slightly audible sound emitted by her before she even begins to speak? What if I realize no one shares my passion or is interested or even gets me?

Big Love: What if?

Me: I'm afraid I will stop believing in myself.

Big Love: Just because one person doesn't get you, it doesn't mean you should give up.

Me: But I know from experience that I don't do well with criticism. I fall apart. It sets me back for days, if not permanently. I am so tired of that negative cycle.

Big Love: Could this possibly be a limiting belief that has outlived its usefulness for you?

Me: Yes ... for sure.

Big Love: What is the worst that could happen?

Me: She doesn't get it and I stop believing in myself ... again.

Big Love: What is the best thing that could happen?

Me: She gets it. She supports me. And my willingness to be vulnerable causes our friendship to transcend to a powerful new level of intimacy. And I have the humility to integrate her suggestions and my project becomes even better!

Big Love: Thank you.

All at once, I realize that I am willing to ask someone to review my project and let go of the results. Talking by phone to Cordelia (50), I'm surprised by the gift of tears. I cry so much I can barely get the words out to ask her, like weird-faced crying, and my voice is all over the place. The tears signify the unmistakable knowledge that this is right. I am healing. My passion is right for me. Whether she gets me or not, whether anyone gets me, I'm ready for the feedback. I won't die; I won't even wither. Her opinion won't cause me to lose my conviction. It will help me express my passion even better. I have picked the right person. I can transcend my limiting beliefs around this area. Crying is truly healing.

Call to Action:
Is there an area around which you are ready to transcend limiting beliefs?

# 307
## WALL PUSHUPS IN PAJAMAS

*Every day I make a self-care contract* for the day ahead, physically, intellectually, emotionally, and spiritually. Some days I am up and at 'em with no trouble at all. I jump into my favorite olive green workout pants, sports bra, and racerback top (green is the new black) and I'm ready to face the day. It is easy to make and keep my daily self-care contract. Other days, not so much. I can barely make it out of bed because the negative self-talk is so mean and convincing.

On those days, I make sure my daily contract is appropriate for that day. I give myself permission to commit to ten wall pushups as my workout ... in my pajamas. No bra. Period.

Dear God,
Give me the ability to discern the caliber of self-care contracts I make today. Because I know how much I love myself by the contracts I make and keep (Patricia Allen, PhD).

# 308

## Physical Balance

*Besides working on spiritual balance,* I also work on my physical balance. One of the exercises I like to do comes from the FallProof Balance & Mobility program, developed by Dr. Debra Rose at California State University at Fullerton.

### Ball Kicking

(Do not attempt if you are unable to stand on one leg for any reason.)

Kick a ball against a wall with right foot. Trap it with left foot.

Kick a ball against a wall with left foot. Trap it with right foot.

Repeat 10 times

Call to Action:
Try a new balance activity today.

# 309
## REFRAMING CONSTRUCTIVE FEEDBACK

*A few days ago,* I asked my friend Cordelia (50) if she would watch my video project for work and give me feedback. I was now willing to risk being vulnerable. It's not like this was the first time I'd risked being vulnerable. And I've had mixed results with putting myself in vulnerable positions in life. But I knew this time was a big deal because I was sharing something I felt very strongly about.

Cordelia assured me she would watch it and get back to me with her feedback. I let it go and went on with my life, recognizing she had a life, too. It was progress for me not to expect her to drop everything and respond immediately, so I was proud of myself. But I noticed something else as well. I was completely calm about the whole thing. I was confident.

For the first time, I got it on a much deeper level that my worth was not riding on her feedback. It wasn't about my worth at all. It was about my willingness and the courage to experience short-term discomfort to allow space for the collective effort of two women to create something exponentially better and more poignant. The day came when she responded. I saw her seven voicemails pop up on my phone. I braced myself not to take her comments personally, as I had in the past when receiving feedback. I sat down with pen and paper to take notes. She gave several thoughtful suggestions. To my surprise, there was not a defensive bone in my body. Her suggestions were amazing, and the thought of implementing them caused me wild excitement. Really? Yes! Imagine that.

I am so glad I was willing to feel temporary discomfort while I let someone see more of me. We both grew as individuals. Equally as powerful was the fact that we also grew closer in our friendship.

Dear Big Love,
Just for today, please give me the willingness and the courage to risk being vulnerable. What if it causes my joy to multiply?

Call to Action:
Consider how you could become vulnerable in one of your relationships today. What if it causes your joy to multiply?

# 310

## HUNGER AND PLANNING MY FOOD WITH INTENTION

*I am grateful to have enjoyed* long-term recovery from an eating disorder for years. I am even grateful for the fact that I have an eating disorder. My perceived and actual appetite are both excellent barometers for what is going on in my head and heart. Sometimes I am unable to discern whether my appetite is actually an accurate representation of my physiological state or I'm having an uncomfortable feeling I am wanting to "stuff down." Making a daily loose plan for my food helps me have the clarity to discern.

Each morning, I think about the 24 hours ahead as it pertains to my food choices. I consider where I will be eating, whether I'll be eating at home, packing my lunch, or eating in a restaurant. If I'll be eating out and know which restaurant, I look up the menu and mentally plan. If I don't know the restaurant, I'll plan loosely which food groups

I'll have, such as a generous portion of vegetables, protein about the size of the palm of my hand, and a carb.

Typically, my loose framework is to eat three meals and three snacks, with the option to have less. The wording "with the option to have less" is specifically chosen because I am a volume eater and I have never been one to skip a meal or eat too little. Depending on where you are coming from, your plan might be worded differently. But basically, I choose these words because we all know that if a recovering perfectionist like me commits to "three meals and three optional snacks" and I end up having the snacks, there is the distinct possibility that my head will then criticize my eating "performance" as unsatisfactory.

This guilty "verdict" could then lead to beating myself up and/or a bout of volume eating. Conversely, if I committed to three meals and three snacks but only had two snacks, I'd have that varsity feeling when my head hits the pillow that night. Building up days of consecutive varsity self-care actions is like putting money in my spiritual bank.

Using this loose food planning technique, if suddenly, I hear chocolate chip cookie dough calling me, I know that is probably not actual physiological hunger. I know that because:

1. It wasn't in my plan (if I did plan to have it, that's another story).

2. It has no nutritional value and creates a physiological detriment within my body.

If it's not physiological hunger, it is perceived hunger. In my experience, beneath perceived hunger is a feeling that I am trying to stuff down with excess food 99-percent of the time. If I put down the food and listen to my heart, answers will come. It may be uncomfortable, but the more willingness I cultivate to listen, the deeper my healing and the more available I am for my Big Amazing Life.

Dear God,
Please give me the willingness to loosely plan my food for today, and the patience to listen to my heart. Help me be brave enough to approach my eating today with intention, so I don't miss the miracles You have in store for me.

# 311

## Costco Hot Dogs, Toast, & Accountability

*As much as I know in my heart* that planning my food and making nutritious food choices to the best of my ability feels best for me, sometimes I am just too afraid to make self-loving food choices. Yes, I have maintained a moderate-sized body for over 30 years. But do you think my food choices and portion sizes have been 100-percent self-loving for that whole time? Of course not! You have to know that there's no way I could have made 100-percent nutritional food choices for over 30 years.

Sometimes I am simply not brave enough to listen to my heart. Something inside me feels too overwhelmed. That's where an accountability partner comes in. The last time we sold our house and prepared for moving day was an example of one such time. The situation called for a lot of people, with a lot of opinions, physical work, and feelings.

With so many moving parts, I was reminded how little control I had over whether my expectations were met. Plus, the weekend that we moved, we experienced weather temperatures in the 90s.

On top of that, I knew that getting all our belongings moved into a new house was only the tip of the iceberg to truly becoming settled in. My nervous system overloaded. There were simply not enough hours in the day. I decided a Costco hot dog would be appropriate and acceptable. And it was. My body doesn't run at its peak on hot dogs, but I was fine with it. I let an accountability partner know and went on with the task at hand.

I think I ate a daily Costco or Wienerschnitzel hot dog and fries and pizza for at least a week during that move … maybe more. I kept being accountable for it and loving myself like crazy. I never gave a thought to weight gain or beating myself up. I embraced what was and knew as soon as I was willing to write about the underlying feelings, my willingness would shift. That is my reality because I am no longer in the diet mentality and have gotten "thin between the ears." I trusted myself and Big Love. Eventually, I found the time to write in my journal to reconnect with my fears. My nervous system calmed down and I happily resumed choosing foods and making choices that better agreed with my body physiology.

Similarly, my friend Cordelia (55) was going through a tough time recently. Her beloved husband had surgery on his spine and there seemed to be one complication after another. On top of that, one of her adult children moved back home for a while. She turned to toast for comfort. I cannot tell you how many accountability voicemails I received from her about her toast consumption. My voicemails back to her said: "Your food is fine. Your weight is fine. I love you no matter how much toast you consume. Give yourself permission to eat toast. When you are brave enough to deal with your present circumstances without toast, you will. Until then ... embrace toast. You will know when toast has outlived its usefulness."

Reflection:
I need to continually remind myself that "cracking down" on my food has never brought me relief.

Call to Action:
Let your food and weight be fine for today.

# 3I2
## NOTHING SHINY IN MY FUTURE

*I've mentioned* that some mornings I wake up with the radio station in my head tuned to KF***. I don't want to go to work, and I don't want to face the day. That's the time when I call my friend Cordelia. I will go on and on about how there's nothing to look forward to. We call it "nothing shiny in my future." I'll move on to talk about how I'm sure I don't know enough to do my job adequately and how today is the day that my imposter status will be uncovered and ridiculed. I will be fired and have no job and soon be living on the streets. It gets to the point where we are laughing. Invariably, she will say, "Do you wanna live anyway, no matter what?" To which I reply, "Yeah, I guess so."

Making the decision to "live no matter what" requires faith and willingness. I have faith that whatever uncomfortable feelings I am experiencing now will pass, even when there is nothing shiny in my future. I demonstrate my faith by becoming willing to make and keep daily self-loving contracts physically, intellectually, emotionally, and spiritually. The tone of each day is contingent upon my faith and willingness.

Dear God,
Help me remember that every day is a beautiful day when I make and keep self-loving contracts.

Call to Action:
Write your self-loving contract for today.
Physically:_____
Intellectually:_____
Emotionally:_____
Spiritually:_____

# 313

## WHAT ARE YOU LOOKING FORWARD TO TODAY?

*Some days I wake up* and my head laments about there being nothing shiny in my future. There are a lot of those days. After all, life isn't Disneyland every day. For people like me who are challenged by unrealistic expectations, tools for attitude adjustment are key. My favorite attitude adjustment tool involves writing.

First, I write a letter to God telling Him how boring my life is and how much happier I would be if _____ (fill in the blank).

Dear God,
Today I am looking forward to spending 10 minutes removing old fern fronds to make room for new fiddleheads.

Next, I ask myself what I am looking forward to today and I reply dramatically, "Nothing, of course!" The point is, I am responsible for my own daily happiness. Therefore, it is incumbent upon me to choose something I am looking forward to every day. There's no other person, place, or thing that is responsible for that.

# 314

## In Search of Fiddlehead Unfurling

*I love ferns.* They are all over my backyard. I am fascinated by the journey of each individual "fiddlehead" of the fern. A new fiddlehead unfurls itself toward the sky to join the existing fully developed fronds to increase the collective beauty of the plant as a whole. Each unfurling fiddlehead reminds me of a human spine as it articulates out of flexion and into a beautiful upright posture. The new fern fiddlehead represents the spine of a confident, courageous woman who is transitioning and articulating into her full upright potential in life. I am so moved by this growth process that I based my business logo on ferns.

My parallels between robust, flourishing ferns and robust, flourishing women continues. Many ferns are so hearty that with the proper care, they can withstand both winter cold and summer heat. With women, it is the same when they take good care of themselves. Both ferns and women need water and the right balance of sunshine and shade.

Every so often, fern fronds turn brown and they look a little withered. But periodic removal of old dead fronds results in a flurry of multiple new breathtaking fiddleheads, stronger and more beautiful than ever. Sometimes as women, we need to remove old "fronds," or beliefs and behaviors that no longer serve us, to make room for newer beliefs and behaviors that better correlate with where we are in life right now.

Something about the sight of unfurling fiddleheads inspires me. It says, "Growth is always possible. Not only is it possible, it is desirable and vital for a Big Amazing Life." My heart is like the fern root ball. When I become willing to look within, in a sense it is like sorting through my beliefs and behaviors to remove those that have become withered. The resulting personal growth is like the emerging fiddleheads: tall, confident, with purpose.

Looking within is hard work that can be uncomfortable. But it prepares my heart to grow and bloom in a new, beautiful way, better suited to where I am in life today. If I don't assess my personal "fern fronds," my heart will become stagnant and wither, never reaching its full potential and full splendor. Looking within through the eyes of nature leads to amazing growth that takes my breath away.

Dear God,
Thank You for ferns. Thank You for speaking to me through nature and ferns. Thank You for growth that takes my breath away.

Call to Action:
What beliefs and behaviors are not serving you anymore? Be brave enough to look within. It may be unfamiliar and uncomfortable. You deserve to have your breath taken away.

# 315
## VISIONS OF DONUTS

*I smelled frying donuts* on my walk this morning as I often do. I fantasized about how lovely it would be to eat donuts with wild abandon. I remind myself I could if I wanted to. I would still be every bit as lovable. I would still love myself like crazy. My family and friends would still adore me. God would still love me so much He couldn't take His eyes off me.

But I would have a stomachache for hours afterward. And my joints would become inflamed from the sugar and the saturated fat. I would probably feel a little like the Tin Man in *The Wizard of Oz* when I tried to move for the rest of the day. And I might have trouble sleeping tonight. I smile and decide to make a more self-loving choice for my breakfast. I always have a choice!

Dear God,
Thank You for giving me choices. I'm grateful to have a choice when planning what I will eat today.

# 316

## DEFINITION OF SERENITY

*Someone told me* the definition of serenity is living with unresolved conflict. I guess I'm not that serene today because all I can think of is donuts. What does thinking of donuts have to do with serenity? Nothing. Everything. The fact that I am romancing donuts is useful information. Let me work backwards to unpack this.

A donut is empty calories, meaning it has no nutritive value. If I am thinking about how nice it would be to ingest something with no nutritive value, knowing the harmful effect consuming it will have on my body, chances are I am not serene. If I am not serene, I am not being willing to accept unresolved conflict. When I look within to discover what person, place, thing, or situation I am not accepting today, I realize I am future-tripping about a huge project for work and wondering if it will be well-received. Will I ever make enough money to pay off my debt? It is impossible to be in the present if I am future-tripping. Therefore, my best thinking told me that having a donut would perpetuate my mental distraction by adding a physical distraction. And adding a physical distraction would further separate me from my God and the people in my life. It's not at all about fear of weight gain. It goes much deeper.

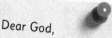

Dear God,

Help me to trust Your plan for my life today, even though it has not completely unfolded yet. Give me the faith to wait for Your next "big reveal" for my Big Amazing Life without non-nutritional food choices. Give me the ability to stay present during unresolved conflict. Thank You for giving me choices.

Call to Action:

Are thoughts about food taking you out of the present? Are you giving away your power and your serenity because you feel uncomfortable? What if it were not at all about weight gain or fear of weight gain? What if it goes much deeper? Are you willing to sit still to discover what is under the surface? Don't quit before the miracle.

# 317
## FEELINGS AND THE
## POWER OF THE PAUSE

*I received an email* from my 93-year-old dad yesterday that has brought up feelings of extreme hurt and sadness. Essentially, we have not communicated since he requested three months ago that I only attempt to contact him if his girlfriend was out of town. At his girlfriend's request, he had closed his bank account and moved all his money to an account I could not access (he had appointed me his trustee years ago), because he suddenly feared I had a secret agenda to "take control of his life and put him away." No amount of persuasion could convince him otherwise.

Does his girlfriend have an agenda? Could she be capitalizing on his highly vulnerable state and exerting undue influence on his decisions? Compelling evidence points to that, but why? I was always nothing but kind to her. After prayerful soul-searching, I rejected the request because it disrespected me. I wished him and his companion every happiness. And. Let. Go.

I thought I had processed the feelings around this situation, and they were "done," like cookies in the oven. After all, I spent quite a bit of time writing, talking, and getting therapy about my relationship with my dad. Wasn't that enough? One more time, I am reminded that feelings don't work that way. I don't get to schedule them, feel them, and put a check mark beside them.

In the email, he reiterated his belief that I desire to take control of him and his money. Anyone who knows me laughs when they hear the outlandish accusation. Still, it hurts like crazy, deep inside to know my own father believes this lie. His mental constitution notwithstanding, it still causes me indescribable pain. Although logically I know it is impossible to determine the origins of his belief, don't think I haven't spent undue hours postulating. My stomach churns and I feel paralyzed and overwhelmed by my current feelings and thoughts. Do I respond? What would I say? I have no idea. That realization makes my stomach churn even more. Peanut butter and crackers only causes the feelings to worsen.

Then I remember the best way to self-care in this situation remains the same. Pause. Take a breath. Step back. Talk about it with a trusted friend. I am grateful I had three people I trust to talk about it with. Write about it. Remember that just because I don't have the answer right now, doesn't mean I am incapable of coming up with an answer. I will trust that answers will come if I stay current with my feelings. I will not die from these feelings. The definition of serenity is living with unresolved conflict. I do not have to resolve this conflict this moment. I went to bed and slept peacefully.

Dear God,
Please fill me with the faith needed to remember answers will come. All I need to do is be willing to identify and feel my feelings and listen for Your answers.

# 318

## Disappointing Others vs. Self-Abandonment

*My dad has been my biggest fan* for as long as I can remember and I his. After he suffered a ministroke, a mysterious abrupt change in his opinion of me strained our relationship beyond measure. The situation has been unbelievably painful for me. Sometimes I feel paralyzed and overwhelmed by these feelings and thoughts. When he occasionally sends an email with confusing mixed messages, it causes me to doubt myself and my self-care decisions around the situation. A voice says, "This is your dad. You MUST respond. The right thing to do is respond! Hurry up! It must be ASAP. Did I mention this is your dad we are talking about?"

At times like this I have learned to affirm, "Thank You, God, for this growth opportunity." I am usually making a face when I say it, but that's okay. Regardless of facial expression, the statement is sufficient to start the healing process in motion … again, but only deeper this time. The growth opportunity has been the ability to come to terms with the extent of my self-abandonment over the course of my life.

I called my friend Cordelia (56) because she is a dear friend who holds a space for me to process ongoing feelings about my relationship with my dad. Additionally, in the past year, we have been experiencing freakishly parallel issues in our lives, even though we have entirely different circumstances. As is often the case, she blew my mind. She shared her latest mantra that was her variation of what Glennon Doyle wrote in *Untamed*: "I would rather disappoint you than abandon myself one more time. I am not willing to abandon myself. Not. Even. One. More. Time. I f-ing love you. I would die for you. But to engage in conversation with you is to abandon myself."

I sit with the thought of disappointing my dad. I compare it with the thought of abandoning myself one more time. Which is more destructive to me?

Dear God,
Please give me the knowledge of Your will for me and the power to carry that out. Thy will be done.

# 319
## POPLARS AND POINTILLISM

*I love poplar trees.* My love for gazing at poplar leaves began long before I knew to take note of things that made my heart sing. My earliest memory of them was in my teens. There was a fancy outdoor shopping mall near my home and the entrance to the mall was lined with a huge semicircle of very tall poplars. I remember loving to watch their delicate, paper-thin leaves quake and flutter freely in all directions in the ocean breeze. It made my heart sing. I don't really know why; I love to watch poplar leaves quaking in the breeze. It's something about the way my brain processes visual events. But if I had to guess, it's something about the way the sunlight hits the leaves as they move freely. The leaves are all moving simultaneously, but independently, in endless combinations that cause a light show of color juxtaposition between the blue sky and the green leaves.

Another thing that made my heart sing was looking at paintings created using the technique known as pointillism.

This technique that grew out of Impressionism was made famous in the mid-1880s by French artists Georges Seurat and Henri-Edmond Cross, among others. As opposed to paint colors being mixed on a palette prior to being applied to the canvas, pure dots of color were applied directly to the canvas. This created an optical illusion of sorts whereby colors could be blended instead by the viewer's eye. Pointillists used different hues of color in combination to achieve this effect. The style depended on the juxtaposition of complementary colors (which enhanced each other's intensity)–such as blue and orange, for example.

Having never considered myself an art connoisseur, I never paid much attention to what happened inside me when I looked at a painting created using the pointillism technique. Sure, I had all the art appreciation modules in elementary school, but I never got why works were supposedly "moving" to people. I usually yawned and wondered how long till recess. However, the only art appreciation modules I enjoyed looking at were when pointillism was the featured painting style. Although even back then, I didn't think much about the fact that I loved looking at them. It wasn't till 40 years later when my son's elementary school did the pointillism module that it struck me. I LOVE this!

I don't know why I love to fixate on poplar leaves and pointillism paintings. Does it matter? Probably not. Both the movement of the delicate leaves and the purposely placed dots of color create a kind of light show that calms my brain. They create a sense of freedom and harmony in my brain. I need to pay attention to these messages.

Dear God,
Help me to remember to pay attention when something is pleasing to look at. These things that make my heart sing. Thank You for things that make my heart sing. Help me remember to seek out more of these things today.

Call to Action:
What makes your heart sing? Try to describe why. Write it down. Seek out more of these things. Listen.

# 320
## FOOD ACCOUNTABILITY

*Yesterday my friend Cordelia* (65) asked me if I would be her food accountability partner. Her weight had once again crept up and she wanted to call me daily to report what she was eating. While I considered my response, I asked her to tell me more about where she'd been regarding her weight in the past few years.

"Well, two years ago I went on a big-name commercial weight-loss program to lose weight for my son's wedding. The weight I lost is now back on, and then some. I just can't bring myself to eat those processed commercial weight-loss foods again so I'm not too sure what to do."

As a health coach, Cordelia's story is one I hear repeatedly. People diet to lose the weight without first taking the time to get "thin between the ears." Meaning they don't explore whether the excess food being consumed is due to emotional eating. And if that's the case, what feelings have been causing them to eat emotionally. Without addressing their ability to emotionally regulate or feel their feelings, no permanent change can take place on their body. The same feelings will continue to fester, having no outlet through which to be expressed. Sadly, I've witnessed countless cases where this endless weight-fluctuation cycle is perpetuated for decades.

Before I was able to let go of the accumulated excess weight on my body for good, I had to completely change the way I thought about and talked about and treated my body. I call this process of mental reconfiguration "getting thin between the ears." For any personal growth to be lasting and permanent, the process of "getting thin between the ears" must precede it.

A lot of people just want the diet. They don't like to hear what I have to say. But I was on my last diet more than 30 years ago. I'm ever so grateful to be free of them! I know firsthand that getting thin between the ears must accompany and ideally precede actual physical weight loss for the changes to be permanent. I inquired if she had considered addressing any feelings she was experiencing. There was an awkward pause. I hate that part. But I allowed the pause and risked her being unhappy with my suggestion, because I have come to a place where I realize it serves neither her nor me to sugarcoat things and tell her what she wants to hear, thereby perpetuating or cosigning for the torturous diet mentality in a fellow human.

I haven't heard back from her and I'm not sure I will. I feel good about not having abandoned myself and what I believe in. Progress! I wish her health, happiness, and a solution that works for her.

Dear God,
Thank You for the willingness to feel my feelings today. They can be scary and uncomfortable, but they will not kill me. When feelings come, please give me the ability to pause in the moment before choosing the immediate gratification food brings. This, too, shall pass. There is no better feeling than identifying and processing a feeling and being on the other side of not having eaten spontaneously.

Call to Action:
Be willing to pause before grabbing food when a feeling arises. Ask God to guide you rather than spontaneously eating. There is no better feeling than identifying and processing a feeling and being on the other side of not having eaten spontaneously. Don't take my word for it. Try it … one time.

# 321

## PC to Apple Computer Learning Curve: Creating New Neural Pathways

*I recently decided* to buy my first laptop computer. Guess I'll be adding "trackpad" to my skillset list. Not only that, I bought my first Apple computer. With all these years as a desktop PC person, I know there will be a learning curve. In the past ten years, I've observed that it takes a little longer to master new things. With those things in mind, I am a little nervous about my decision.

Yet the growth opportunity that comes with the presence of these new variables is precisely why I made this choice. Although I know inevitable frustrating times lie ahead, it's vital that I continue to constantly create new neural pathways in my brain as I age. Creating new neural pathways in my brain helps me let go of old self-limiting beliefs that no longer serve me.

One of the self-limiting beliefs I am working to let go of is that if I am not fast enough and competent enough and smart enough, I will be deemed obsolete and unlovable. Each new trackpad "gesture" I practice, slowly master, and memorize smashes that lie I believed about myself and is replaced by the "I am Varsity-Caliber Lovable and Capable at any age!" belief. All is well.

Dear God,

Thank You for the willingness to try new things. Thank You in advance for the self-patience I'm gonna need as I embark on this new experience. Remind me I don't have to be the best and the fastest at navigating my new computer. I don't have to nail it by noon today. I am very much still lovable in every case.

# 322

## FIND & FOLLOW EXUBERANCE EVERY DAY

*Merriam-Webster's Dictionary* defines **exuberant** as joyously unrestrained and enthusiastic.

In Marc Brackett's *Permission to Feel*, he shares: "Joy and exuberance produce more feel-good neuro-chemicals such as serotonin and dopamine, which help us

Dear God,

Thank You in advance for more serotonin and dopamine secretion today! As for my part, today I will keep my senses poised for things to be joyful and exuberant about. The touch of my Vizsla Wilson's buttery soft fur. The calls of local California quail, Nuttall's woodpecker and the house finch who gently pull me out of my future-tripping head and bring me back to the present moment. The promise of new fiddlehead ferns unfurling. Eye contact with my son.

direct our thoughts where we want them to go. We then also secrete less cortisol, the stress hormone, if we are practicing some small morsel of joy and exuberance every day."

Call to Action:
Initiate some serotonin release today! Using your five senses, find one example of exuberance in your day, with the option for more. Write it down. What is it?

# 323
## Ten-Minute Laundry Folding Challenge

*It's that difficult time of the morning* where I cannot bring myself to get into the shower. Thoughts of all the unknowns and "what-ifs" I face today and just in general leave me paralyzed with fear. There are a lot of changes in my life right now. How will I handle them? How will I cope? Will I make the right decisions? Am I present enough for my child in this phase of his life? Is there anything I need to do differently? What if I am missing out on some opportunity due to my shortsightedness? I know my thoughts and fears are a little over-the-top and somewhat irrational, yet I am unable to rein them in.

On my way to take out the trash, I pass by the laundry and remember there is clean laundry in the dryer from yesterday. I stop and spend 10 minutes folding it. For some reason, the act of stopping to fold laundry brings me back to the present. In my head, I redirect all the questions and self-doubt. I remind myself I don't have to have answers to all these questions right now. Today is a day where I need to keep it simple. My job is to move my body in some way that brings me joy, get in the shower, choose self-loving foods, and portion sizes to the best of my ability and show up for life. The rest is in God's hands.

Dear God,
Help me remember to keep it simple today. To determine my three top priorities today and then leave the rest to You.

# 324

## YOU ARE WORTH THE TIME REQUIRED FOR FOOD PREP

*I've mentioned before* I consider myself a former volume eater … whole cakes, pies, pizzas, loaves of bread, sticks of butter. When it comes to choosing self-loving foods and portion sizes 75-percent of the time, I have found there are three secrets:

1. Planning ahead (both mentally and with the action of food prep).

2. Keeping good-tasting, and at least somewhat nutritious snacks readily available.

3. Prepare in bulk, place portions in individual baggies, and freeze whenever possible.

Yes, that takes extra work. But nothing beats that feeling of knowing there is something special in that fridge waiting for me that won't leave me with a food hangover.

I was unable to locate the source of this recipe. I received it about five years ago from a lovely woman in my Pilates circuit class in Long Beach and I make it often. The original recipe also called for ½ cup of goji berries. Because I keep hearing conflicting reports about the nutritional value of goji berries, I usually don't include them these days. The recipe is excellent with or without them.

Food Prep Call to Action:
## No Bake Chocolate Almond Oat Bars
    1 cup brown rice syrup
    ½ cup coconut oil
    ½ cup almond butter
    ½ tsp sea salt
    2 tsp vanilla
    2 tsp cinnamon
Heat the above ingredients in saucepan over low heat. Remove from heat.

Chop dry ingredients below (except for the chocolate chips) to desired consistency:
    1 cup chopped almonds
    1 cup chopped walnuts
    ½ cup sunflower seeds
    ½ cup pumpkin seeds
    2 cups rolled oats

1 cup dark chocolate chips

Add chocolate chips to saucepan and stir in. Then stir the rest of the dry ingredients into the saucepan. Press into greased 9" x 14" cake pan and refrigerate until hardened. Cut into 32 bars. [Recipe can be halved]

# 325

## HOT VEGGIE LOVE IN A MUG

*Many people extol the benefits* of banning certain foods or food groups. They believe that banning foods is the only answer and proclaim it to anyone willing to listen. My journey has been a bit different, as I have found it far more beneficial to focus on which foods I eat than on which foods I refrain from eating. The food choice journey in me honors the food choice journey in you.

In my 20s, once I determined and embraced the fact that volume eating tends to be my default to cope with anxiety, I set out to compile a list of the best foods to consume in quantity. Naturally, vegetables topped the list. From that epiphany on, I approached each upcoming meal by first choosing which veggies it would contain. Additionally, the veggies are typically the first part of my meal that I eat. This habit buys me some time to discern between my actual physiological hunger and any emotional hunger I may be experiencing at that moment.

One of my favorite veggie recipes is Collard Green Soup. This soup not only fills me up physically, but also just makes me feel loved. I cannot say enough good things about this recipe or about Abbie Gellman, RD. Not only are her recipes packed with nutrients, they are also freaking delicious, different from the norm, and easy.

Food Prep Call to Action:

**Collard Green Soup**

(Double this and Freeze!)

Adapted from a recipe by Abbie Gellman, RD

> 1/8 – 1/4 cup olive oil
>
> 1 yam or celery root (or half yam & half celery root),
>     cut into squares (skin on, if using potato)
>
> 1 yellow onion, diced
>
> 3 cloves smashed garlic
>
> Salt to taste
>
> Red pepper flakes to taste
>
> 2 boxes veggie broth
>
> 1 bunch Kale (lacinto or other)
>
> 1 bunch Collard greens
>
> Lemon zest of 1 lemon or to taste
>
> Juice of half lemon
>
> 1 bunch parsley

Add garlic to salt. Strip stems off kale and collard greens.

Add olive oil plus potato/celery root, onion, cloves, salt, and red pepper flakes to large pot. Deglaze with half cup of stock. Cook until the liquid is reduced by half.

Add greens, rest of stock, and bring to a boil, then reduce heat to medium, cover and simmer for about 25 minutes or until greens are tender.

Remove from heat. Add lemon and zest to Vitamix. Puree soup with lemon/zest till blended. Add the parsley into last batch.

# 326
## CROCKPOT CHICKEN

*Making nutritious food choices* is, in general, more expensive than making non-nutritious food choices. For example, a package of organic turkey runs about $6.00 and only yields about two servings. Do you know how many bags of sour cream and onion potato chips you can get for the same price? Luckily, there are ways to cut costs. One thing I do regularly is buy an entire chicken for about $10.00; less if I watch for sales. It takes about ten minutes of prep time and then 3-4 hours to cook in my crockpot while I go on with my day. Once cooked, I discard the skin and freeze the carcass to make bone broth for Wilson later. The refrigerated protein easily lasts for the week. Simple and delish.

Dear God,
Thank You for the World Wide Web and the willingness to try new things. Help me remember that while food prep takes a little extra time and forethought, the resulting feelings of self-value and well-being far outweigh the investment.

# 327
## Hummus

*Many people liken overeating to alcoholism,* believing that banning certain foods is the only solution. They label their food plan "Clean Eating."

I don't argue that certain ingredients, such as, sugar offer virtually no nutritional benefit and can cause inflammation, especially in a perimenopausal or menopausal body. Nor do I disagree that, when consumed in large quantities, even more physiological and mental issues can arise. The problem with the food-banning mindset and the "Clean Eating" label is that they are not realistic. If I expect myself to "eat clean" or never to eat sugar, I set myself up for failure. No one can eat that way 100-percent of the time. Hell, even ketchup contains sugar. When that inevitable time comes when I consume sugar, my brain perceives failure. And with that perceived failure comes a barrage of negative self-talk that I would never wish on anyone and then what? Am I "dirty?"

My journey has been a bit different, as I have found it far more beneficial to focus on foods I do eat rather than on foods I refrain from eating. As I like to say, the food choice journey in me honors the food choice journey in you. With that in mind, I also like to choose foods that complement foods that I eat the most of. Hummus is an example. The flavor of my beloved vegetables can be enhanced when dipped in hummus. Thus, eating hummus incentivizes eating more nutrient-dense veggies. Hummus for the win!

### Easy Hummus Recipe

(Better Than Store-Bought) by Adam and Joanne Gallagher. It can be found on their website: www.InspiredTaste.net.

Makes 6 servings or about 1½ cups

YOU WILL NEED:
- 1 (15-ounce) can chickpeas or 1½ cups cooked chickpeas
- 1/4 cup fresh lemon juice (1 large lemon)
- 1/4 cup well-stirred tahini
- 1 small garlic clove, minced
- 2 tablespoons extra-virgin olive oil, plus more for serving
- ½ teaspoon ground cumin

Salt to taste

2 to 3 tablespoons water

Dash ground paprika or sumac, for serving

DIRECTIONS:

In a food processor bowl, combine the tahini and lemon juice and process for 1 minute, scrape the sides and bottom of the bowl, then process for 30 seconds more. This extra time helps "whip" the tahini, making the hummus smooth and creamy.

Add the olive oil, minced garlic, cumin, and a ½ teaspoon of salt to the whipped tahini and lemon juice. Process for 30 seconds, scrape the sides and bottom of the bowl, then process another 30 seconds or until well blended. Open, drain, and rinse the chickpeas. Add half of the chickpeas to the food processor and process for 1 minute. Scrape sides and bottom of the bowl, then add remaining chickpeas and process until thick and quite smooth; 1 to 2 minutes.

Most likely the hummus will be too thick or still have tiny bits of chickpea. To fix this, with the food processor turned on, slowly add 2 to 3 tablespoons of water until you reach the perfect consistency.

Taste for salt and adjust as needed. Serve hummus with a drizzle of olive oil and dash of paprika. Store homemade hummus in an airtight container and refrigerate up to one week.

Call to Action:
Are you willing to try something new? Be sure to buy veggies when you get the hummus ingredients!

# 328

## WEIGHING THE PRICES AND PRIZES OF FOOD CHOICES

*Sometimes I just want a cookie,* the kind with truly little nutritious value. The kind with ingredients that can cause inflammation on my precious hormone-level-challenged joints. And I always have the option of having one. I have a choice. Typically, I plan a dessert day about once a week. First, I choose some dessert that I deem to be a "10." Then I either buy it or make it and thoroughly enjoy it. Then I get on with my Big Amazing Life.

Other days, if I really analyze it, I realize I don't necessarily want an actual full-blown cookie. I just want something that looks like a cookie. Chews like a cookie. Smells like a cookie. Handles like a cookie. I want to hold it in my hand like a cookie and enjoy it. But I don't want the joint inflammation. I want to feel good physically, emotionally, and spiritually, above all else. On days like that, I make peanut butter granola bars from my *Forks Over Knives* cookbook. As always, I double the recipe, cut into portions, and freeze in individual baggies.

Dear God,
When food cravings come, please give me clarity about what I want. Is it worth the cost to my body? Is it worth the inflammation? Or would a reasonable facsimile work just as well?

# 329
## CRACKER POWDER & COVID-19

*I am grateful* for my eating disorder because it serves as a barometer for me. When I find myself unwilling to make self-loving food choices, I know I need to look at my spiritual fitness for that moment. I am most likely having feelings which I am unconsciously trying to avoid. Yesterday was one of those days. My first awareness that maybe I was not spiritually fit came as I stood in the kitchen, consuming a large bowl of granola, mixed with half & half that was two days past its expiration date and a golf-ball-size chunk of brown sugar, followed by the pouring of bottom of the box saltine cracker "powder" straight from the box into my backward-tipped head.

When I went straight from those actions to mentally contemplating making a cheese and mayo sandwich, I realized I might be having a feelings issue. I called my friend Cordelia (56) to reveal the snack I had just consumed, to which she replied, "I freakin' LOVE you!" We both laughed and then she sweetly asked, "Are you having some feelings?"

I knew she was right. After I made and consumed my cheese and mayo sandwich, I sat down to write. As always, my writing brought awareness to feelings I had not been in touch with. I realized I was quite anxious about my COVID-19-influenced financial situation. About two weeks prior to COVID-19, I had been laid off from one of my jobs. Then with COVID-19, I became 100-percent unemployed. I was in a lot of fear.

Then flattening the curve took much longer than originally anticipated. Next, the introduction of the various stages of workplace reopenings during COVID-19 made determining when a health coach should return to work perplexing for me. When would be the safest time for me to return to work? Was I considering all the variables for me and my family? How could this timing possibly work out? Was my career pivot going to be a viable move for me?

Dear God,

Help me remember when I am afraid that I am trying to visualize a solution with my finite brain, rather than Your infinite power. Please remind me that I am not able to see how this timing is going to work out. And remind me to believe the outcome will be outstanding, like nothing I could've ever imagined. Because I'm not God.

# 330
## COVID-19 & UNREALISTIC EXPECTATIONS

*I am constantly reminded* of my endearing default of unrealistic expectations (UEs). And each time my affinity for UEs, as I call them, shows up, I am caught off guard. How cute am I? COVID-19 was no exception. There I was, proudly quarantining, feeling like a boss. After about four weeks of it, I had gotten in the swing of it and felt surprisingly good. I stayed home, worked hard, and visualized the day when we received the "Curve Completely Flattened" declaration and I could return to doing things my way again.

Yes, I had frequently heard the expression, "the new normal" but for whatever reason, I hadn't understood the full implication of what that meant. Again, it was my UEs default in action. I excitedly was waiting for the time when we would receive the green light to leave the house at will, shop without fear of being mask-shamed, and hug each other with wild abandon.

Imagine my shock when I discovered there was a 4-stage resilience road map published by *Covid19.ca.gov*. At the time, we were just entering stage 2, which gave a green light for lower-risk workplaces to reopen. Nothing else changed. Leaving the house still had restrictions, masks were still very much in the picture, and wild-abandon hugging was still way off in the distance.

One more time, I needed to right-size my expectations.

Dear God,
Thank You in advance for another huge dose of open-mindedness, faith, and willingness to seek and do Your will today. Thank You in advance for the ability to let go of my UEs ... I crack me up.

# 33I
## IF I'M KIND TO ALL PEOPLE, COULD I STILL BE RACIST?

*For the past several days,* news stories about the *Black Lives Matter (BLM)* movement and protests against racial injustice and police brutality have spread across the US and beyond. This is not the first time in my life that stories such as this have made headlines. Unfortunately, it may not be the last. As usual, I get uncomfortable hearing them. It saddens me deeply to hear that another black person lost his life for absolutely no reason. Stories of looting and violence preempt normally scheduled television programming. Scared and uncomfortable, I turn off the television.

As usual, I run through my mental checklist about my concept of racism that goes something like this: Am I racist? … of course not. I am kind to everyone I meet. I look all people in the eye when I speak to them. I decide who I want as a friend, based on my observation of a person's character, not her skin color. I'm good. I will just stay quiet for a while until this blows over.

I check social media. Several posts make me uncomfortable yet again. While I don't remember the actual comments posted, what my brain perceives is: "If you make no comment on the situation, you are racist. If you do nothing, you are racist. If you are silent, you are racist."

Now I am even more uncomfortable. Is this accurate? Am I, in fact, racist? And if I am, what can I do about it? I let myself sit with these uncomfortable white fragility feelings for the day.

> *Dear God,*
> *Am I racist? I thought I wasn't. I don't want to be racist. What can I do? Please guide me. Thank You for humility. Thank You for the willingness to deepen my understanding of the definition of racism.*
> *Love, Sally*

> *Dear Sally-Girl,*
> *Well, let's say you look at racism as a scale. Would you be willing to explore where you are on the scale? Having awareness of your ignorance is a good place to start. I love your willingness to be uncomfortable, as well. Let's do the work.*
> *Love, God*

# 332
## BEING TEACHABLE

*As Black Lives Matter sentiments* continue to flood social media, I continue to cry spontaneously, not even exactly sure what I am feeling. I continue to pray about and ponder my participation in this movement. I have a mom friend who is black. Our sons have been friends since fourth grade. Like many mom friends, we have fallen out of touch as our kids' interests have become more varied. I consider calling her. That would be weird. Will she be offended at my calling out of the blue? Will it be uncomfortable? How would I start the conversation? I decide to call anyway, not at all sure what to say. I dialed my friend Cordelia (41). Like old school call: it is 7:15 a.m. on a Tuesday. She picks up groggily, "Sally?" I start to cry. I don't even know why. It doesn't matter. I tell her I want to learn. If she wants to talk, I want to listen. It's uncomfortable. It's painful. It's healing. I am glad I called. Hearing her perspective helps me better understand. It occurs to me that for me to be an anti-racist, I first need to be self-confident enough not to take it personally when someone expresses huge overwhelming feelings. Thank you, Cordelia, for holding a space for me to unlearn and learn anew. I'd like to be able to hold a space for you as well.

Have I stopped racial injustice by making this call? No. Have I made a significant difference? I don't know. It is a baby step. And it is a baby step in the right direction. I am no longer worried about whether people label me as racist. Maybe I am racist. But I am teachable. The first step is not shutting down when I read things that make me feel uncomfortable. I can learn more. I can ask questions. I am willing to learn how to be an anti-racist.

Dear God,

Give me the confidence to sit with my uncomfortable feelings long enough to be able to hear the feelings of black people, and all BIPOC (Black, Indigenous, [and] People of Color). As with all feelings, my own and others', it is not my job to fix them. Please use me in a powerful way, one day at a time. I am open.

# 333
## PAUSING & PROCESSING

*On my journey to explore uncomfortable feelings* around racism, the discomfort continues. Today my discomfort comes from the fact that I suspect my friend Cordelia (59) has unfollowed me on social media. We have been friends for over 10 years. She hasn't returned my calls lately. I'm starting to wonder if it has something to do with my recent posts in support of the *Black Lives Matter* movement. Ordinarily I wouldn't give this much thought, but for some reason this morning it's taking up a lot of space in my mind. I am willing to learn how to be an anti-racist.

I find myself going to my default, which would make one of us wrong. I want to take immediate action to stop these unpleasant, repetitive voices in my head. I rehearse various imaginary conversations with her. I want to yell at her, "What's wrong with you?" That doesn't feel right. I consider taking her temperature, "Will you still be my friend if I believe in this?" That doesn't feel right, either. It becomes evident that as usual, I'm worried that, if I am completely myself and talk about my opinions, I will wind up with zero friends—lonely, unlovable, and alone. My own personal journey here is once again, am I willing to be me and let people see that … even if it means losing friends? I inwardly smile and realize that my answer is a resounding yes.

I call another friend who is pretty much on the same page with me on this issue. She reminds me that I am processing, and I may need some time and space to do that. And that I will process this the same way I process everything … over time, with journaling, and with prayer. She reminds me that my friend is also processing, and she may also need some time and space to do that. And it may look completely different than what my processing looks like. That reminder causes a long sigh as my shoulders relax.

Oh, yeah. One more time I remember it takes time for all of us to process new information. I do not have to act immediately. For today, I am willing to sit in the uncomfortable unknown, trusting and respecting that we are all doing the best we can.

Dear God,
Give me patience and understanding as I figure out my beliefs and opinions. Please also give me patience and understanding for my friends and their beliefs and opinions.

# 334
## STILL PROCESSING

*I continued to wrestle with* the suspected social-media unfollowing situation between a friend and me. "Should I flat-out ask her if she unfollowed me?"

"What would I even say?"

"If she says yes, should I ask her why?"

God, please give me knowledge of Your will for me and the power to carry that out. Please use me in a powerful way.

I continued to call her every day for several days in a row. My calls went to voicemail. Finally, I texted her, saying she was on my mind. She called me. We talked for quite a while about the normal things we talk about. I couldn't come up with words to address the topic of racism.

The next day, her posts were showing up in my feed again. Could it be that she was following me all along but had gone silent from June 1-7? ... maybe. Could I have done a better job handling that phone conversation? ... maybe.

Could I have brought up my allyship journey? Could I have shared with her my support of antiracism? Yes. Instead, I exercised my white privilege prerogative by failing to bring up the uncomfortable topic, thereby conveniently ignoring it so as not to risk conflict.

This situation raised my awareness and made me think. I want to do better. I am constantly looking within to be a better human. The area of racial equality is no exception. I am willing to do the work. I am willing to imperfectly, uncomfortably keep trying.

The imperfect allyship journey in me honors the imperfect allyship journey in you.

Dear Big Love,
I am still listening.
I am still learning/unlearning.
I am still growing.
Give me the courage and the words to say to open those uncomfortable conversations about race. Any friend who I lose in doing that was not my friend to begin with.

# 335
## White Saviorism

*My imperfect allyship journey continues.* Social media posts by multiple BIPOC (Black, Indigenous, and People of Color) suggested that non-BIPOC support black businesses. Eager to listen, learn and grow, I began to follow black people in the field of wellness and mental health. I learned about a virtual course on antiracism. I was so excited about the course I connected with the course creator and asked if she was offering the course to a large national organization on wellness. She said it was in the works. I asked her if it was okay for me to contact the organization to inquire where they were in their course inclusion process for a large upcoming event. I love connecting people. She said yes. I sent a couple emails passing on the course information. I was excited. Including the content at such a large event seemed like a great way to impart valuable, timely information on a huge scale.

Later that day, I perused the resources glossary from the book *Me and White Supremacy* by Layla F. Saad. My stomach sank when I came to the term white saviorism. Was my attempt to connect going to be perceived as merely an act of white saviorism? Immediately I called my friend Cordelia (50) and related my story. She assured me that doing nice things for people is just who I am. Still unsure of how my gesture would be perceived, I realized I had to let it go. The business owner had every right to her opinion. I could check my ego and stop trying to explain and defend myself.

I'm still super uncomfortable at times. I don't have to take her temperature to see if she is mad at me. Am I willing to be an imperfect ally regardless? Yes. I have never truly been an ally before. How would I know how to be one? I will only learn by taking action. Despite my discomfort, this feels right. Thank You, God, for this opportunity to heal from my impression management and people-pleasing.

The imperfect allyship journey in me honors the imperfect allyship journey in you.

Call to Action: Risk appearing imperfect. Risk being a novice. Just say something.

Dear Big Love,

I feel frustrated. It seems like every way I turn, I am criticized. But help me remember that a lot of the time that critical voice is coming from within me, not from outside. Help me remember my goal is not to be praised by anyone. My goal is to come from love instead of fear.

I am still listening.

I am still learning/unlearning.

I am still growing.

# 336
## TIMING

*Lately I have been fearful of financial insecurity.* What if I cannot support myself as I age? What if I must resort to a job I am overqualified for, and that I dislike? What if I must work at this job until I am 80 years old to survive? And even at that, I am barely scraping by? But even bigger than that is the fear that I will never reach my full potential in life because I was unwilling to walk through fears. I was unwilling to believe in myself and follow my heart.

When I hang out in fear, I am in the future. I remember, I have enough for today. I remember I am not in charge. I remember I am future-tripping using my finite human brain, rather than trusting the infinite plan of a bigger picture … of Big Love.

Dear Big Love,
Please help me trust Your timing. Could You please send a reminder about how perfect Your timing is? I know You gave me some amazing examples of Your perfect timing about two months ago, but I can't remember what they were because of my CRS (Can't Remember S***-Stuff). I promise to keep my eyes open today.

# 337
## Emotional Literacy in Action

*I received a voicemail* from my friend Cordelia (40) yesterday. She is one of my most spiritually grounded friends. She rarely uses profanity. In fact, in the 7+ years I have known her, I can probably count on one hand the times she has dropped an F-bomb. At the same time, she is completely accepting of the semi-regular full-blown expletive-laden voicemail rants I leave on her message center. I treasure this friendship.

This voicemail was quite a departure from her normal even-keeled manner. She prefaced the message saying she was experiencing what I call the "KF***" mindset as opposed to KJOY mindset. She used several choice expletives to describe her frustration at the time of the call. She began by citing lack of sleep and a clingy toddler who had inadvertently done the classic top of head lift/slam into Cordelia's bottom jaw. From there, mom cried out in pain, beginning the domino effect of child crying, leading to parent guilting.

Cordelia continued. Uncontrollable schedule changes in her business brought about by current world events and the seeming inability to get anything on her "list" completed. I believe she dropped more swear words in that one voice-mail than she has over the entire time I've known her.

Was this radical behavior shift fueled by shifting hormones? … perhaps … perhaps not. The point is, if you possess the skill of emotional regulation, you have a better chance of navigating the twists and turns of life while simultaneously self-cherishing. Cordelia is emotionally literate. She possesses the skill of emotional regulation. When she experiences uncomfortable feelings, she expresses them in an appropriate way, in a safe place. She got a babysitter and went for a drive. She left a voicemail to express feelings. In talking aloud in the message, she realized her feelings of frustration. Further, she identified that her frustration about her inability to complete her intended "list" for the week was triggering her addiction to "efficiency."

Now Cordelia went a little deeper and voiced her feelings of extreme sadness, confusion, and hopelessness about the racism brought to light by the *BLM* movement. She realized and reminded herself she needed to give her feelings to God with a willingness to participate in the solution, although she had no idea of what that might look like. To trust that if she watched and listened, she would be guided. She became willing to let go of her timing and accept all these circumstances as God's intended, perfect timing, and all this in less than three minutes. Impressive!

Dear God,
Please give me the willingness to sit with uncomfortable feelings as I await Your guidance about my next indicated step. Give me the ability to trust that I can do all things in You who strengthens me. My job today is to express my feelings in a healthy, normal, and appropriate manner while I self-cherish to the best of my ability. And wait.

# 338

## SEASONS OF LEARNING: A KINDER/ GENTLER TERM FOR OBSESSION

*I love discovering new things* to learn about. Life constantly presents opportunities for learning. I call them seasons of learning. When a particular learning season grabs my interest, I tend to get fixated on it. I research multiple sources on the topic, with gazelle-focus. It consumes me. I visualize different versions of it. I dream about it. I wake up in the night thinking about it. I want to talk about it with my family and my friends. My appetite for learning about the season is seemingly insatiable. I simply cannot get enough information about that season. Addictive personality much? So lovable.

Seasons have woven together throughout my life, making me the person I am today. It is not uncommon to have two different seasons overlapping. Seasons vary in length from months to years. Some seasons last decades or even a lifetime. For example, in my 20s when I began my recovery from an eating disorder, it was a season of learning how to eat, combined with learning to love my body and learning about communication skills. When I gave birth to my child at age 40, a long season of parenting took shape. When my son turned six years of age, I continued with the parenting season and I became fascinated by learning everything I possibly could about the mind/body practice of Pilates. Then there were the seasons of beading/bracelet-making, gardening, and mosaic creations.

This characteristic is an attribute and a good thing if I keep things in perspective. Bottom line, through this process of information uptake and sorting, I decide which people's stories resonate for me. Which people's journeys will I adopt to become a better version of myself? Which people's philosophy will I emulate to help make the world a better place? My seasons concept is one of the ways I redirect my addictive personality in a positive direction.

Put in the simplest terms, "one could say that long-term recovering from addiction or overcoming any defect of character you are unable to conquer on your own, requires recovering from extremes with a reliance on a power greater than yourself." It is a lifelong, one-day-at-a-time journey to restore balance and perspective in every possible area. The foundation of my personal journey is built on embracing wherever I am on that spectrum on any given day, without judgment. From this vantage point, I have been able to move through the extremes and find the balance for over 30 years.

So, circling back to the "seasons" concept, my newest season is becoming an anti-racist. Achieving balance and perspective within a season requires first letting my thoughts and emotions run the gamut without judgment. This season is no different, although it is right up there with some of my most uncomfortable seasons. On my information-gathering journey, I have become willing to inventory my part in systemic racism. I have become willing to explore racist beliefs mirrored by my parents. I have listened. I am reading recommended books on becoming anti-racist. I have connected with more black people on social media. That is super exciting for me, as previously I had wanted to but feared rejection. I have reposted their posts. I will continue to connect. I have had uncomfortable conversations with both white friends and black friends. I will continue to act as I learn more.

On my feelings journey, I have felt defensive, angry, and afraid. I have shamed myself and felt shamed by others. I have self-judged. I have judged others. I have felt judged by others. I have felt like both the persecutor and the victim. I have felt like I am to blame for all of racism (extreme much?). I have felt incredibly sad, depressed, overwhelmed, and hopeless. It is heavy. In short, I have allowed my thoughts and emotions to run the gamut without judging myself or others. And this was all in one week.

Dear God,
Help me remember that I will make sense of all these thoughts and feelings. Help me remember it will take far longer than one week. My current season of becoming an anti-racist will be a lifelong season. I'm listening. I'm in. Make me a channel of Your peace and love.

# 339
## COVID-19 & CLARITY

*Since I tend to be overly self-critical,* sometimes I mistakenly blame myself in a situation where I have done nothing wrong. Thankfully, I know this about myself and take a regular look at my behavior to examine my part. This practice brings me clarity and keeps me from unnecessarily blemishing myself. Of course, there are times when my action has been inappropriate, and I need to acknowledge that. Regular inventories keep me current in all my affairs.

Several times during the COVID-19 experience, I heard the question asked, "How have your values changed as a result of the pandemic?" Each time I heard the question, I had a new awareness. The pandemic helped me pinpoint relationships that no longer served me. Not only that, relationships that possibly had never served me. Yet prior to global sheltering-in-place, I had not listened to the inner voice that softly said, "Why are you in that relationship? You don't feel good when you interact with that person. You don't feel supported by that person. Why do you continue?"

Taking a closer look, I began to beat myself up for staying in a relationship for literally years that was almost completely one-sided. It helped me to journal about my part in the relationship and my feelings. Then I remembered, "Gentle, gentle." Next time the person contacted me, I set a boundary that I was busy and unavailable to talk. Her texts persisted, demanding to know more about why, ignoring my boundary. At first, I felt awful for not responding. I berated myself for that behavior as well and then I journaled some more. Again, I remembered, "Gentle, gentle." I held my ground. I am not sure why I have difficulty putting my self-care needs before the needs of some people, but I am willing to look at it and am making progress. Today I realized that I misinterpreted this situation. For whatever reason, my default is always that I have the problem. My boundary was healthy, normal, and appropriate. The person was not honoring my boundary. What a feeling!

Call to Action:
How have your values changed lately? Write down one way, with the option to write more.

# 340
## SELF-CONFIDENCE NOSEDIVE

*As I became ensconced* in my new lifelong season of becoming an anti-racist, the rush of feelings became so overwhelming, I found myself consumed by depression. Yesterday I was so depressed that I was paralyzed, unable to comprehend the reality of the lives of black people for so many years. For days I had cried and allowed myself to feel the feelings, but in time it crossed the line because I had internalized it too much and it rendered me unable to do my job. I decided to go for a drive. I ended up at the produce market. In the parking lot, I got out of myself by texting my friend Cordelia (40). She is the friend who's a single mom of a toddler who had the pervasive KF*** situation a few days ago. I inquired if she needed any groceries.

Getting out of myself always gives me perspective. When I delivered her groceries, we had a socially-distanced conversation about my anti-racist journey. My mood was somewhat lifted. I realize that, little by little, I will find the balance in this new season. I will determine my role as an anti-racist and be confident in it.

Dear Big Love,
Please give me patience as I embark on this day. Give me knowledge of Your will for me and the power to carry that out.

# 341
## CORDELIA'S REVELATION

*After having had some time* to process information about the *BLM* movement, Cordelia feels compelled to dive in.

First reaction: "Oh no, I cannot take any more sadness." Second reaction: "I feel inspired and ready to fight on behalf of equality. I hope this time we can make history."

Dear God,
Your guidance will give me the strength and courage. I'm listening.

# 342
## SORTING OUT COMPLICATED FEELINGS

*I have been working to get out of credit-card debt* for just over a year. The process is slow, but I am focused and not finished. I have an agreement with my former husband that we will not use a credit card without first discussing it with each other. Yesterday, as my son was leaving to have dinner with his dad, he informed me that his dad had been paying for their last several dinners out with a credit card.

Fueled by anger, I grabbed my phone and dialed him, asking if our previously-agreed-upon spending terms had changed (knowing full well that they had not). Historically this approach has not worked because it causes him to become defensive, thereby reacting with anger. Yet I let myself act spontaneously. The result was predictable and the conversation unpleasant, with accusations flying both directions with an abrupt ending. My son left and I was alone with my feelings.

I called a friend and left an unedited lengthy voicemail outlining (spewing) my feelings. Then I wrote a letter to my former husband and one to God.

The next day my son and I sat down to discuss the previous day's situation. He had considered his part and decided this was all between his dad and me, and therefore did not have his name on it.

I owned up to my part for letting him be in the middle of an issue that didn't involve him and apologized. I marveled at my son's emotional literacy. I marveled at our ability to sit down and calmly discuss an emotionally charged situation after the fact.

Dear God,
Thank You for the knowledge that I can go back and review uncomfortable interactions after the fact. Thank You for the tools that enable me to communicate with the people in my life. Thank You for the willingness to look within at my part in each interaction and own my part within myself, with You, and with others involved.

Call to Action:
Are there any previous interactions you have had with others that you could revisit and clean up?

# 343

## LISTEN TO YOUR COMPASSIONATE VOICE

I've recently begun hosting an Instagram Live Event I call Varsity Midlife Pivot, where I interview women about their life journey amidst the pandemic, their career, and aging. What challenges they've faced and how they've made sense of the challenges and persevered. The response has been positive. Yesterday I became more vulnerable and began the event with a guided meditation. Today when I found that my food choices and amounts for lunch consisted of an entire 7.5oz. bag of Trader Joe's Vegetable Root Chips and most of a package of "Brookies" alternated with chunks of cheese, I knew there were some feelings going on. A redirect was needed … I decided it was time for my CV/CV writing exercise.

*My Critical Voice:*

*Dear Sally,*

*That was really lame yesterday on Varsity Midlife Pivot. You have all of three listeners. You are so not an expert on meditation. And you spoke way too fast. Everyone was bored and uninspired. What were you thinking? Who do you think you are? While we're on the subject of your performance in general, you should just give up on your pandemic career pivot. No one is interested and no one cares, and you will never get things off the ground to make a career of menopause coaching. Hah!*

*My Compassionate Voice:*

*Dear Sally-Girl,*

*I am so proud of you. Your Varsity Midlife Pivot Events are powerful on multiple levels. Your agenda to empower women to share their stories and therefore inspire themselves in the process really resonates. From there, that message reverberates to every woman listening. Although your listener base is small, feedback has been overwhelmingly powerful and 100-percent positive. Consider the percentages. That was only your second time to conduct a guided meditation using social media. That was coura-geous. You can practice and improve on your meditation delivery. Keep going! Keep doing what you are doing. You have a purpose. The world desperately needs you to utilize your motivational gifts. Stop playing small. Don't waste another second doubting yourself.*

*Always remember, God loves you so much He can't take His eyes off you!*

Call to Action:
Is there an area of your life where you have been playing small? You know you have gifts that you haven't been utilizing because you are listening to your Critical Voice. What would your Compassionate Voice tell you? What are the gifts?

# 344
## SHIFTING FROM DREAMING TO BELIEVING

*For over 15 years,* I have dreamed of working with women to help them navigate menopause. There have been many, many times when I gave up my dream because I got too scared. I would listen to the lies my head told me. I would become overwhelmed. One more time I would decide to ignore my dream and repeat what was familiar. Granted, the familiar hadn't worked in the past, but at least it was familiar. None of my friends really got what my vision was, either. When I would try to verbalize it, their body language spoke volumes to me, and I would retreat into my shell and vow not to speak about it again. After a while, I stopped talking about my dream to anyone. For years I prayed for guidance. I prayed to find someone who could help me make my dream a reality.

One day while having iced tea with a relatively new friend, Cordelia (46), we were talking about our career aspirations. Against my better judgment, I shared a little about my dream. She actually "got" my idea. Her support was so enthusiastic, in fact, that at first, I discounted her opinion. That's how much self-doubt I was filled with. With time, however, I have allowed her genuine enthusiasm to permeate my psyche at the cellular level. From that point on, I have relished the opportunity to speak to Cordelia about my dream. Whenever I speak about it, she goes wild with excitement. Her level of support, encouragement, and conviction is compelling.

Cordelia sees in me something I can't quite see in myself.

Reflection:
I am grateful for Cordelia ... for she believes in me. I need to let her know how much her support has enabled me to shift from merely dreaming to believing in my idea. After all, she "gets" me!

Call to Action:
What is your dream? Is there someone who "gets" your vision? Seek that person out.

# 345

## SHIFTING FROM BELIEVING TO DOING

*I have mentioned* my unstoppable vision of working with women to help them navigate menopause. And I have mentioned *ad nauseum* how many times I have given up my dream because I was too fearful about anything unknown or new. Every time I tried to discard the idea forever, the Universe just kept bringing it back to the front of my brain. Has this ever happened to you?

Praying for some sign that the idea had merit, I met Cordelia (46) who was a huge supporter. Her support spurred me on as never before. As supportive as Cordelia was, she was not able to physically help me bring my idea to fruition. I prayed more. I searched for the right type of mentor or coach who could help me determine actual action steps. I kept getting "No." Nothing came, so I continued with my "day job."

I landed a day job I had wanted for years. I thought this job would lead me to where I wanted to go regarding my career vision. Things were going well. They were not going in exactly the direction I had been hoping, but the clients and the people I worked with were incredible. Plus, I was learning valuable new skills. I vowed to stay open-minded and to work hard for a year and see what developed. I met many remarkable people while working at this job and it was an enriching experience for me.

My favorite person was Cordelia (28). She was 30 years my junior, young enough to be my daughter and then some, but we somehow clicked. I kept thinking about my maturity level when I was 28. I let my insecurities go. I even dared to talk about my menopause coaching idea, never expecting a vibrant 28-year-old woman to get something like that. She told me nonchalantly that she could help me with implementing my ideas, but at the time, I didn't think much of her comment. Maybe she was just being polite?

Then after six months on the job, Cordelia and I were both suddenly and unexpectedly laid off. No real explanation, but we were both given glowing letters

Dear God,
Thank You for Cordelia. You really were listening. Please continue bringing me support for my dream even though I have no idea how it could possibly come to fruition.

of recommendation. Letters of recommendation notwithstanding, we both still had shock and deflated egos to embrace. We still had resumes to update and interviews to land.

We stayed in touch and helped each other come to terms with our respective unexpected change-of-career plans. It was invaluable to have each other to lean on as we rebuilt our confidence and planned our pivots. We met for coffee to talk about our resumes and respective job searches. BTW: Resumes have really changed since the 1980s. Again she casually mentioned she could help me. It took a while for me to become willing to let her words sink in ... but thankfully I did. BEST DECISION EVER!

Cordelia's positivity and nonstop encouragement were invaluable. She saw for me something that I couldn't quite see for myself: My dream could become a reality! Not only that, she saw it BIGGER than I could see it. She was the person I had prayed for.

Call to Action:
Have you ever given up hope about your dream because you could not envision every single action step required? Keep believing. If your heart knows you are meant to do this work, thank God in advance for support with your dream. And thank God in advance for bringing you just the right people to help you.

# 346

## Awards & Focus

*My friend Cordelia* (50) left me a voice text requesting an award. We often request an award from each other when we have accomplished something we consider noteworthy. An award consists of either a cell phone text containing an emoji of a trophy, or a verbal proclamation of the word "AWARD!" … or both. It is unbelievable how satisfying this small thing feels. It often thwarts a bout of spontaneous eating, and never results in a stomachache, painful joint inflammation, or insomnia the way spontaneous eating can. It doesn't take much to make us happy.

Cordelia wanted an award because she had stayed focused on a task from 9:30 a.m. to 2:00 p.m. She was ecstatic about the fact that she could stay focused for so long. I could hear it in her voice that she was over the moon. I immediately voice-texted her at the top of my lungs: AWARD!

Understandably, she was eager to determine the reason for her prolonged, uncharacteristic ability to focus. I smiled as I listened to her entire recorded message. She rattled off possible variables in hopes of replicating the freaking focus "formula." Her variables included: food combining—just the right ratio of beets to cacao; hours of sleep; exercise; meditation, or Self-Myofascial Release. Although these were all quite possibly responsible for her stellar focus, I knew all too well about the unpredictability of hormonal shift. Thankfully, my only job was to acknowledge my dear friend with an award. I stayed inside my own hula hoop.

Dear Big Love,

Thank You for awards. Remind me to give myself permission to ask a friend for one when I deserve it. Meanwhile, please give me the ability to enjoy the peaks and valleys of my day. Give me the ability to soak in the joy during the peaks and trust the process during the valleys.

Call to Action:
Have you asked anyone for an award today? Give yourself permission to ask.

Have you given anyone an award? You can even give an award to a stranger in the grocery store. Try it!

# 347
## Dismantling Mindsets: part i

*The topic of systemic racism* has come to my attention in a big way. I am reading books to educate myself. I am listening. I have been warned I will feel uncomfortable, and I do. I am doing the work anyway. Today I took a course about anti-racism to learn more. The more I look within to examine where I am in my thinking about a racism mindset, the more I uncover about myself. The more I realize how much I don't yet understand, the more I realize how much work there still is to do.

Looking within to learn where I—as a person of white privilege—fall on a racism scale is new for me. However, I am no stranger to looking within. I am no stranger to doing uncomfortable work on myself. I have done so for over 35 years. There are a few other mindsets I am always working to recover from. They no longer serve me, so I work daily to heal from them. I have added "racism mindset" to my list of mindsets I'm actively working to heal from. When any of my identified mindsets reveal themselves, I take it as a sign that more work needs to be done. I need to create new neural pathways through commitment to new behaviors on a sustained, daily basis.

Dear God,
Please give me the courage to look at where I fall on the racism scale to heal from this faulty mindset. Then give me the ability to learn new neural pathways that dismantle my racism mindset.

Call to Action: What are you doing to become anti-racist?

# 348
## DISMANTLING MINDSETS: PART II

*One of the ways I stay in fit spiritual condition* is to explore which mindsets are no longer serving me so that I can take contrary action to become a better human. I do this type of exploration on a regular basis. Most of my faulty mindsets stem from the character defect of perfectionism. I have long referred to myself as a recovering perfectionist. Perfectionism Mindset shows up for me in three main categories:

*1. Impression Management:* This means I attempt to manage your impression of me by carefully choosing which parts of my life I reveal to you. This is a mindset that originated in my childhood partly because of a message I received. The message was: Look good at all costs. Look perfect. Be the expert on whatever you talk about. Show this version of yourself to the world because if others knew the real imperfect you, they wouldn't love you, accept you, or even like you. And they would judge you and hurt you.

As if I could control anyone's impression of me. I have an unrealistic expectation of myself that says I am only lovable if I am perfect. The self-expectations are about everything from body to thoughts to what my house looks like, and everything in between. Impression management is exhausting on every level. The truth is, I am at my most lovable when I show up flawed. I have heard true intimacy defined as me being me and letting you see me.

2. *Explaining and Defending*: This mindset stems from the belief that I am not a valuable member of society unless I am perfect. My worth is inextricably linked to my performance: If I make a mistake, then I am worthless. Therefore, my value is constantly at stake. This mindset makes it virtually impossible for me to own my part in any situation. Instead I attempt to pivot the blame onto someone else, anyone but myself.

3. *People Pleasing*: This mindset stems from my belief that if you disagree with my opinion you won't love me and, therefore, I am unlovable. In the past, I have tended to be nice all the time, thinking I am controlling your opinion of me. I will read your body language and twist myself into a pretzel to become the person I think you will like the most. The truth is, if you don't like me because we disagree on

something, I don't want you as my friend. Not only that, we were never friends in the first place. I have come a long way in recovering from this.

These mindsets are areas I will work on for the rest of my life. Now that I have begun to look at where my behaviors and thoughts fall on the racism scale, I see how the perfectionism mindset hinders my journey to dismantle racism.

Impression Management tells me to remain silent on the topic of racism because I am not an expert. I am willing to let that go.

I am also willing to let go of my white fragility which manifests itself as "Explaining and Defending." I am willing to change my behavior.

Dear God,
Open my mind to listen and learn today. Help me let go of striving for perfection. Open my mind to healing from a perfectionism mindset and be willing to create change within myself to create change in the world.

People Pleasing tells me not to voice my opinion on controversial topics for fear of making people uncomfortable. I am willing not to waste my time worrying about that anymore.

This newfound awareness gives me even more reason to learn new mindsets. There is no place for perfectionism in anti-racism. To quote author Layla F. Saad, "Create change in the world by creating change within yourself."

# 349
## GETTING OUT OF BED AWARD!

*Dear Sally-Girl,*

*I know you woke up depressed today. Today was one of those days where it seemed there was nothing shiny on the horizon, yet you mustered the strength and courage to get out of bed. Given all the uncertainty you face in your life today, I'm impressed. I know you have been working tirelessly and there is seemingly little to show for it. But you got up anyway. I know you like awards. Give yourself a Getting Out of Bed Award today. You have true faith and belief in both Me ... and in you.*

*Way to go! Do not give up. The goal is in sight; you will get there. Some days will be harder than others to believe this, but keep believing anyway. Don't quit before the miracle. Answers are coming, even answers on tasks you've no idea how to solve right now. Be patient. Continue to self-care and do footwork while waiting for answers. I love you so much I can't take My eyes off you. Love, Big Love*

# 350

## SELF-CARE DURING
## UNRESOLVED CONFLICT

*I have two legal issues pending* in my life right now. There is a legal form to be completed and submitted. There are emails to respond to. I don't know all the answers required to complete the form, so I cannot respond to the email. Additionally, I will need to contact an attorney and an accountant, among other professionals to address the issues.

Issues involving the law or attorneys, and income taxes or accountants are not my strong suit. I am not an expert in these areas. The reminder of those facts heightens my stress and anxiety. I want to eat spontaneously over both issues. I am having a lot of negative self-talk around how each of these issues will be resolved. I just want it all to stop.

I ask myself, "What self-care will make me feel better right now?" Rationally, I know both issues will get resolved, but just not today. That knowledge does absolutely nothing to assuage my extreme physical and mental discomfort. I revise my question, "What will the footwork toward the solution look like for today? How will I live with unresolved conflict?"

Living with unresolved conflict is one of my greatest challenges to date. I review actions I have taken today so far. I have contacted "people" and am waiting for their responses. I have eaten all the hummus-dipped veggies I can take and licked the hummus container clean. I have opened the fridge several times, but neither God nor a magic insertable "legal knowledge" computer chip seem to be in there. I have refilled the bird feeder in my yard. I have called a friend to identify the extreme anxiety and depression I am experiencing today. I have called another friend to get out of myself by asking how she is doing today. I pray. I ask God for guidance. The unpleasant feelings remain. I decide to look at the legal form again. I reread it, this time it makes a little more sense, but I take a deep breath, realizing it still will not get completed today. I made self-loving food choices, watched mindless television with my son, and went to bed. The definition of serenity is living with unresolved conflict.

*Dear Big Love,*
*Please give me the ability to live with unresolved conflict*
*without excess food today. Help me remember that there*
*most certainly will be a corresponding high to match the*
*lows I felt today.*
*Love, Sally*

*Dear Sally-Girl,*
*Great job on footwork for today. I am so proud of you*
*for rereading that form that seems overwhelming to you.*
*AWARD!*
*Love, Big Love*

# 351

## Do the Footwork & Trust

*When I awoke today,* I asked God for guidance. Next, I checked in with my body and feelings. Not all, but a significant portion of the anxiety and depression I experienced yesterday was gone! Yes, my two legal issues still loomed. But the fact that I had imperfectly chosen self-loving foods and amounts the day before had had a huge impact on my sleep last night; a huge impact on how my body felt this morning; and a huge impact on my feelings this morning. All the above were significantly improved. And getting out of bed this morning took much less persuasive self-talk than yesterday.

The two legal issues from yesterday are still unresolved, but my anxiety over them is reduced considerably. I was on multiple conference calls with not only a historically difficult person, but also an attorney and an accountant. I did all right! I didn't know all the answers, but it went okay.

Today I can see that things are moving in the right direction and my patience is renewed. Breathe ….

As a former volume eater, eating is my go-to. I embrace that about myself. Over the last 30 years, the healing I have had in this area is nothing short of a miracle. To a large degree, I attribute my healing to my willingness to stop dieting and completely re-configure my thought process around food.

Dear God,
One more time, thank You for the reminder that for every low, there will always be a corresponding high to match it. I need only be patient.

# 352

## ACCOUNTABILITY PARTNER & BOOKENDING

*Yesterday I called Cordelia* (50) to bookend her. A bookend is where I tell another person I trust how I am feeling. In this first of two bookends, I identified the extreme anxiety and depression I was experiencing. I put it all on her voice-mail: all the feelings; all the irrational fears; all the negative self-talk; and all the future-tripping. I also included all my catastrophizing and every example of my scarcity mindset *du jour.*

Then I walked uncomfortably through my day imper-fectly, without padding my food to quiet my busy mind. I just suited up and showed up for the day, even though I didn't want to, and even though I was mentally paralyzed with fear. Bookending is a tool I use with my friends to help me through hard moments. It didn't matter that we didn't have a live conversation with each other. I knew she would listen to my voicemail. Knowing another person knew my state of mind was immensely comforting.

Today I left her another voicemail. I call this the second bookend. This is the follow-up to the first bookend to tell her I lived through the tough time. To tell her how much better I feel and how much calling her helped. The tool of bookending serves several purposes. It helps remind me I am not alone. It reminds me this feeling/situation/negative self-talk, too, shall pass. It reminds me that every feeling has a beginning, middle, and end. No matter how much it seems permanent in the moment. The second bookend is confirmation of that. Bookending gives me faith in myself. Bookending keeps me accountable. Additionally, bookending cultivates all the above with both me and the friend I call. It's a win-win.

Dear God,
Thank You for my friend Cordelia. I'm grateful to have a safe, nonjudgmental friend who holds a space for me to process my feelings.

# 353
## What Am I Thinking?

*The other day* I was at the grocery store. Not the huge warehouse-type grocery store, but just my normal local grocery store. I couldn't help but notice they now offer not only the double-sized bag of chocolate chips, but also an even bigger size. The law of supply and demand tells me if this size is now available, there must be a demand for it. Why would that be? I'm certain it is because people must be doing some emotional eating right now. Times are uncertain. I get it. I eat chocolate chip cookies sometimes. There's nothing wrong with that! To understand where I am coming from, I need to back up a little.

I regularly take inventory of my thoughts. I think some negative things sometimes. I use several techniques to change my negative thoughts. I practice gratitude, I do service, I do specific writing exercises in a journal, to name a few. I don't take these actions because they are super fun. It takes discipline to take these actions. I take these actions because I know that my thoughts influence my emotional health. And my emotional health influences my physical health. If I don't practice intellectual and emotional self-care, I tend to make non-nutritious food choices.

Practicing emotional regulation for me means identifying, feeling, and expressing my feelings. If I don't stay current with my feelings, I tend to eat spontaneously in ways that don't feel good physically. If I make non-nutritious food choices, I don't feel good physically. I continue to have even more negative thoughts, which, in turn, impact my emotional health more. I continue to make non-nutritious food choices to the extent that it harms my body and impacts my body's ability to function optimally. And around and around it goes.

Dear God,

What I weigh is Your business. What I do with my thinking is mine. Help me remember to do my part. Please give me the willingness to stay current with my thoughts and feelings in healthy, normal, and appropriate ways.

# 354
## Fat-Shaming Male Gynecologist

*When I was about 12,* my mom took me to her gynecologist for my first visit. It was the early 1970s. There I was, supine-lying and stirrup-footed. The doctor leaned over me and grabbed an entire handful of excess skin to one side of my navel and asked shamingly, "What is this? We need to do something about this!" I was understandably mortified on several levels. I was super-young and vulnerable. It was my very first visit to a gynecologist. He was male. I was raised to view medical professionals as the authority on all things. Therefore, my takeaway was this: He is right. I am overweight. I am unlovable. I must lose weight or men will not be attracted to me. I should be ashamed of myself for eating in a gluttonous way that has caused my body to be disgusting.

I never told my super-thin mother about it because I suspected she might have even phoned ahead to ask the doctor to say something about my body. I feared she would take the side of the doctor anyway about the fact that I needed to lose weight. She was the one who put me on my first diet at 10 years old. I never told anyone about this doctor's comments until 20 years later because I was so ashamed. My reasoning was it wasn't "that bad." I had heard stories of women having been raped by doctors, so I should just keep my mouth shut and be grateful that's "all" that happened to me.

Oh, by the way, while I was never one of those super-skinny kids, I was well within a healthy weight range for a young woman approaching puberty. The whole experience was outrageous and sad. This event, coupled with the fact that my well-meaning mother put me on a diet at age 10, set in motion a decade of believing lies about my lovability and

Dear Big Love,
Thank You for continuing to heal me from my experience with a medical professional. Help me to continue to value myself, my lovability, and my body the same way You value me.

my worth, and the relationship of both to my body size and shape.

Thankfully, I have focused my intention on healing in a major way and have made amazing progress in the 40+ years since then. My story in these pages is a testament to that. The healing and growth continue today.

On the bright side, I've had three wonderful male gynecologists care for me over two decades. And then I realized I could choose a female gynecologist!

# 355

## Permission to Listen to Your Gut

*After the bad experience* with the male gynecologist's fat-shaming comment in my youth, I continued to be seen by that same doctor until I was about 18 years old. Looking back, I am incredulous this was the case, but considering I never told my mother about the doctor's comment, why would she think there was a need to find a new doctor? And since it had been my first gynecological visit, I just assumed this was what could happen. Prior to the time of the visit, I had been binge-eating in private and had had extreme shame about it. Therefore, I readily bought into the lie that I was defective because I secretly ate such large quantities of food. The doctor's comment only served to reinforce the lie. Thankfully, the Universe stepped in and that doctor eventually retired.

After my first gynecologist retired, I saw three more male gynecologists over the course of 20 years, including the one who delivered my son when I was 40 years old. All three were excellent.

It took me a while to give myself permission to really listen to my gut. Still unaware, the Universe again stepped in. When I was in my early 40s, my then-doctor retired and my insurance assigned me to a female gynecologist. I clicked immediately with this doctor and except for one brief period, she has been my doctor ever since. Unfortunately, she moved two hours away a couple years after we met. My gut said it was worth it to drive the two hours required to continue seeing her. My head said it didn't want to drive all that way. At first, my head won. There must be someone else nearby.

On the recommendation of a friend, I went to another female doctor, hoping we would click in the same way. We didn't. Although she didn't touch me inappropriately or shame me, I sensed she shared the same diet mentality my original male doctor

> Dear Big Love,
> Thank You for the constant gentle reminder that I am worth it and for giving me permission to listen to my gut.

had had. That was when I listened to my gut and began driving 2-2.5 hours for my annual female checkups. I'm so glad I realized I am worth it.

Call to Action:
Do you love your gynecologist?
You deserve to love her or him.
Give yourself permission to listen to your gut.

# 356
## VITAMIN D WALKING

*As an all-or-nothing kind of gal,* balance is always a challenge for me. I'm the type of person who wants to work on one project for hours on end with no interruptions. Part of this mentality stems from the fact that once my hormones began to shift, staying focused became increasingly difficult for me. If my head was thinking about one task and I was interrupted, it created two time-consuming challenges. For example, if my son asked, "Can I throw this dressy shirt in the washer with my load of jeans?" the first challenge would be to wrap my head around his simple question. Then, the second challenge would be to resume whatever I had been doing before his question. The whole thing could take 20 minutes or more.

One of the ways I deal with this is by taking what I call a Vitamin D walk. When interrupted, I take it as a sign I need to take a break and switch gears. I get outside and walk around my block. It only takes about 10 minutes or less. I take deep breaths, lift my chest, and walk tall. I swivel my hips. I take in the vital nutrients from the sunshine on my face, arms, and legs as I walk. As hard as it is to believe, taking a break stimulates my brain and makes it easier for me to resume what I was working on. What was it again?

Dear God,
Please help me give myself permission to take breaks every 20 minutes or so. Increase my faith that I will be able to resume and that I will accomplish "enough" for today.

# 357
## Learn by Doing

*Because of a cell phone service glitch,* I am still able to see one of my son's (now aged 20) email accounts on my cell phone. Due to my short attention span that I've already written about *ad nauseum,* I have never taken the time to correct the glitch. Today I noticed he received an email reminder from his auto mechanic about when his car needs to be serviced.

Without a thought, I opened a new text to him, asking him the mileage on his car. The "human doing" in me wanted to get right on this, even though the service wasn't recommended for at least a month. I stopped myself. Wait! This is his car, not mine. I am doing him a disservice if I micromanage this. I delete my empty text bubble to him. I mark his email as "unread" and exit his email. I went on with my day. I did, however, go out to the garage and check the mileage on his car and compare it to the mileage noted on the email. Then I really went on with my day. But still this is huge progress for me, and I give myself an award. Me compared to me, I'm amazing. AWARD!

Dear God,
Please give me the ability to let my adult son handle his own affairs. Please give me the ability to let this go. Help me remember if he is to become a capable adult, he needs the opportunity to learn by doing.

# 358

## THE INTERSECTION OF BODY ODOR, BRAIN FOG & SELF-FORGIVENESS

*Ever since my hormones began to shift,* body odor has been an issue. Apparently, this is universal, as evidenced by the huge response I get whenever I ask other women about it. The discussion swings from sweating in new body regions, to deodorants/antiperspirants tried, to which laundry detergents can remove odors. I've been feeling good about using Native deodorant for about a year now. But I've not yet found a laundry detergent that can remove odor from my clothes. I've even had to throw clothes away.

Just when I feel as if I have tried everything, I'll hear something new. Recently, my friend Cordelia (52) suggested trying the laundry detergent called Persil. You can imagine I scoured the laundry detergent aisle next time I was at the store. I even had my son looking. We could not locate this product called Persil. We completed the rest of our shopping and began checking out. Suddenly, two check stands down I spotted a large blue container of Persil in a woman's cart. "There it is! They do carry Persil!" The astute grocery bagger asked if I'd like him to get some Persil for me. He came back shortly with three choices: the high efficiency; the odor-remover; and the spot-remover versions. Of course, I chose the odor version. As if that wasn't enough excitement, the checker then pointed out that I could use a $5 coupon from my receipt toward the purchase of the detergent. I practically floated out of the store on the way to my car I was so excited. My son quietly asked, "Did you know none of the detergents the man brought you were Persil?" "WHAT? Why didn't you say something while we were in the store?"

"I did but you dismissed me."

"I did? I am so sorry. I didn't realize THAT'S what you were saying."

I vaguely recalled my son had been saying something while I was choosing which bottle of detergent, but this was one of those times when brain fog rendered my processing time either extremely slow or nonexistent. The bottles were all blue. And the brand name began with the letter "P." WTH? Whatever the case, I am the proud owner of a huge blue container of NOT Persil. At least it is the odor-release formula. I'll keep you posted if it does the job.

*My Critical Voice:*
*Dear Sally,*
*You are so stupid. Can't you read? Pay attention! Listen when your son speaks to you! Your parenting skills are awful. Now you have wasted money on yet another product that probably doesn't even work. You MUST go right back into the store to exchange it.*

*My Compassionate Voice:*
*Dear Sally-Girl,*
*What an honest mistake. You are human. Your parenting skills are exactly right. Pandemic grocery shopping is overwhelming to begin with. Wearing the mask makes your glasses fog up, partially blocks the reading portion of your lenses, and challenges your balance. Plus, you were trying to process conversations with the amazing checker and grocery bagger simultaneously. It was just too many variables at one time. You are human and adorable. Give yourself permission NOT to go back in to exchange the item. How about you just try the product!*

*Always remember, God loves you so much He can't take His eyes off you!*

# 359
## MOM'S ATTEMPTS TO MOLD ME

*Growing up with two older brothers,* there was a distinct disparity between the way my brothers were parented and the way I was. As a young girl, my mother would stress the importance of eating like a lady. She had an extreme preoccupation with my thinness at any cost, as if eating was a moral issue and thinness equaled purity. I envied my brothers because at dinner they could go back for seconds or thirds without scrutiny. To make matters worse, during the warm summer months, my brothers could hang out in only their cutoff shorts, without wearing a shirt. Up until a certain age, I relished hanging out with them in identical attire. I clearly remember when my mother informed me I was no longer allowed to do that. From then on, I would always be required to wear a top, even though my brothers could do whatever they pleased. It seemed as if they had all the freedom and power. For that reason, I was a devout tomboy, probably even beyond the age where this was developmentally appropriate. It just seemed like being male was where all the power and freedom was.

So naturally, I disliked my mother's attempts to mold me into her concept of what I should be. The mere thought of acting like a lady was repugnant to me. The thought of eating like a lady was worse, if that's possible. I came to feel ashamed of my ravenous appetite. Acting like a lady sounded like restraining my true personality, as if there were something inherently wrong with it. Consequently, I took on the belief that something must've been wrong with my body because I was required both to restrict what I fed it and keep it covered up.

After considerable work on myself and guidance from therapists, I have been able to appreciate where my well-meaning mom was coming from. I have released her with love, knowing she did the best she could with what she was taught by her own mother and her mother's mother and so on. I love her dearly and cherish memories of taking night-school sewing and calligraphy classes together when I was a teenager.

Working through issues in the relationship with my mom enhanced my ability to heal. I was finally able see that the journey to better physical, intellectual, emotional, and spiritual health had to begin with loving my shape exactly as it was. My diet mentality fell away, and I gave myself permission to eat whatever I wanted. I fell in love with my body and made peace with food. I finally felt as free as my 5-year-old me had perceived my brothers to be.

That was only the beginning. The next work was uncomfortable and imperfect, and progress was slow. It required a sustained daily commitment to what I call Extreme Self-care and Self-love. I don't always like it, but I do it anyway because I always remember my Why. I fall in love with every part of ME, every day, down to the cellular level: my thoughts; my feelings; my imperfections; my idiosyncrasies; and my irrational fears.

I came to these realizations over thirty years ago. I still practice them (imperfectly) every day. Join me.

Dear God,
Thank You for another day of willingness to learn, grow, and heal, no matter how uncomfortable I am.

Call to Action:
Be willing to commit to Extreme
Self-care and Self-love every day.
You don't have to always like it,
but be willing to do it anyway.
Remember your Why. Be willing
to fall in love with every part
of you, every day, down to the
cellular level: your thoughts; your
feelings; your imperfections; your
idiosyncrasies; and your irrational
fears.

# 360

## MINDSET CREATED TO PERPETUATE RACIAL INFERIORITY: FAT PHOBIA

*As a girl*, I remember my mother stressing the importance of controlling my voracious appetite to "eat like a lady." Although I was young, even then I knew this thinking was bizarre and wrong. I wanted to please my mother, so I outwardly acquiesced. Yet inwardly, I rebelled. So began a 14-year journey of rebellion in the form of disordered eating and body dysmorphia. Thankfully, I have worked to overcome the fear-based, limiting beliefs imparted to me as a child and have gratefully enjoyed a shame-free relationship with food and my body for many years.

I am admittedly late to this conversation, but I am grateful to be having it now. In May of 2020, the *Black Lives Matter* movement got my attention. On my journey to become anti-racist, I began reading to dig a little deeper. One booked was especially helpful: *Fearing the Black Body: Racial Origins of Fat Phobia* by Sabrina Strings, PhD. It helped me understand where my mother's beliefs came from. The book traces racially motivated historical developments as early as the Renaissance period. A mindset was purposely created to perpetuate racial inferiority. This mindset gained momentum and eventually led to the fear of fat and glorification of thinness currently experienced in the United States.

Strings' book articulates what I knew intuitively as a young girl: my mother's and this country's obsession with thinness and dieting was/is wrong. But there is even more to it than I had realized. The perpetuation of disdain for overweight female bodies stemmed from an attempt to create race, sex, and class hierarchies that degraded black women and disciplined white women. My eyes are opened. My work continues.

I especially recommend this book to any woman committed to doing her own work to become anti-racist, who has ever shamed herself (or judged others) because of an imperfect body, eating habits, or both. I also recommend this book to any woman who refers to eating habits as "good," "bad," or "clean."

To think that the origins of fat phobia date back to the Renaissance is incomprehensible, and even more compelling because there is so much that needs to be dismantled. There are far more important things to consider than the number on a scale. Now is the time.

Dear God,

I feel sad to learn about my ancestors' treatment of people. Please guide me as I sort through this information and examine my white privilege. Use me in a powerful way as I unlearn with my eyes open. What is Your will for me in changing my legacy and changing the world? Thy will be done.

# 361

## Last Conversation With Dad

*I will always remember* the last conversation with my dad. On a Tuesday he was taken to the ER for an abnormally high blood pressure reading. His symptoms were stroke-like, although the presence of his pacemaker made it impossible to confirm a stroke. By Friday, the hospital was ready to discharge him to a nursing home for two weeks to monitor his progress. Remembering his mantra—*if you put me in a nursing home, I might as well drive myself off a cliff*—I knew it was time to connect with him. I called Saturday. He was not able to hold the phone by himself and I could barely make out his words. Because the parameters around the pandemic prohibited me from physically visiting him, I had to accept that knowing he knew it was me calling was enough.

The next morning, I called again to see if I could hear any improvement in his voice. He sounded like someone whose mouth was still numb from a dental appointment, or he had stuffed cotton balls in his mouth. With continued patience and repetition, I learned to decipher what he was saying to some extent. I understood enough to realize that he was more coherent than he sounded. And without a doubt, he was tracking what I was saying. I even got the chance to mention one of our favorite family shows, *Get Smart*.

I asked him if it was time to make arrangements for him to come home. He emphatically replied, "YES!" I assured him I would begin immediately when we ended the call. Most importantly, I told him several times how much I loved him and that I understood why he had done what he did, forbidding me from seeing him for the last six months of his life. His repeated "I love you, too" were loud and clear.

> Call to Action:
> Have you made peace with your parents? Now is the time.

We ended our call and, as promised, I called the hospice nurse who had cared for my mom seven years earlier. Who is this woman? Who remembers me from seven years ago and will speak to me for 54 minutes by phone on a Sunday? Rose will. On that call, we arranged for an emergency hospice determination the same day and planned to bring my dad home.

In less than an hour, I received word from the nursing home that Dad's heart had stopped beating and he was gone.

# 362
## Dear Dad

Dear Dad,

*Saying goodbye sure is hard.* Thank you for all the happy memories, laughter, and love.

Childhood memories I cherish:

- Laughing together when you put Oreo cookies inside your glasses.

- Watching *Get Smart* with you.

- Riding to the car wash with you on Saturdays, always sitting on your briefcase so I could feel as tall as you.

- The sound of your wingtips on the tile floor when you arrived home from work each evening.

Thank you for always believing in me.

Jim Blackburn

3/16/1927 - 8/23/2020

# 363

## Dear Dad From Me in Five Years

Dear Dad,

*I feel peaceful.* I've forgiven you completely. And I've forgiven the person involved who verbally bullied and intimidated you into alienating your daughter for the last six months of your life.

All that is left are the fun, happy memories and laughter with you, Mom, and our family. The great father you were. The house on the street where you lived is gone from my life. I'm a fully functioning, free adult, now doing the best I've ever done in every area of my life. Fully alive and free. I can't wait to see what the future brings next. I will love you forever and picture you happy, reunited again with Mom.

# 364

## GRIEVING AND GRATITUDE

*Today my brother,* my son, and I met at the jetty at 7:00 a.m. to honor Dad. We were informed by the cremation organization we worked with that our dad's ashes would be scattered two miles out from the end of the jetty. Dad was in the navy during WWII, and all his life he loved the ocean. He loved swimming and boating, and this was one of his favorite places to go to gaze at the ocean. Unfortunately, the organization refused to provide us with a window of time when we could see the boat. At first, they wouldn't even disclose the date of the scattering, because that would've been a massive up-charge from the original $1,600. While we couldn't narrow down a time, with some authentic waterworks, I was able to persuade them to at least give us a date.

It was about an hour and a half of sitting together and getting to know the brother I really have never known all that well. Death brings unexpected surprises. Death heals some things.

While the three of us sat on the bench, a persistent hummingbird repeatedly returned to the flowers directly before us. It was a beautiful setting. Gazing at the Pacific Ocean as the backdrop, we recounted how Dad loved his hummingbird feeders and how he delighted when one would come to the feeder just outside his kitchen window.

I don't know what you believe, but somehow, I felt this Allen's hummingbird was Dad's way of telling us he knew we were there to honor him. And he would have been thrilled that my brother and I were finally getting to know a little more about the last 40 years of each other's lives.

Eventually we were all talked out. We collectively decided to designate the next boat to come through as "Dad's" boat. Fittingly, the next vessel to come through the jetty was named *Nautilus*. According to Merriam-Webster.com, nautilus is from the Greek *nautilos*, meaning sailor. We silently watched as the *Nautilus* made its way out of the jetty at 4.4 knots, into the vast Pacific Ocean.

Reflection: Grieving and gratitude lead to acceptance.

# 365

## HOLDING A SPACE FOR GRIEVING LOSSES AND GRATITUDE

*I've covered the importance of gratitude.* Gratitude leads to acceptance. Most of the time, it takes discipline for me to get into gratitude. Yet, I willingly do it because the benefit is so great. It changes me for the better on every possible level.

Lately I've been learning the importance of grieving. Not my favorite pastime, I've tried to avoid it if possible. Thank you, Big Love, for this growth opportunity. I would even venture to say that for whatever reason, this last six months has been a super-sized season of grieving losses.

As with all loss, there have been chapters ended. There have been chapters ended by the Universe and those ended by me. I've grieved the loss of my father, my second marriage, and even friendships. Of those chapter endings initiated by me, those took great amounts of courage to consider what was in my own best interest as the top priority.

I've also grieved about things that didn't even happen within this self-defined grieving season. My mother died seven years ago but since the recent loss of my dad, it seems natural to grieve my mom again on a deeper level. I have jewelry of hers that my dad gave me when she died, and I have kept it wrapped up all these years. I just wasn't ready to look at it. Until now. Yesterday I was able to unwrap it and lovingly go through each piece. I'm wearing a necklace of hers right now and I remember her dearly.

I honor the importance of allowing a space for grief as a natural part of life. Even daily, if needed. As a natural part of healthy aging. Some of the ways I grieve are through hearing, writing, and crying, or a combination of all three. For me, the sound of certain piano music can elicit almost instantaneous response if my tear ducts need expression. I allow that space for a few minutes each day during turbulent times.

Just as grieving is imperative, so, too, is gratitude. The day after my parents' home of 30 years was cleared out to be put up for sale, I awoke at 3:00 a.m. with a heart so heavy that it was palpable. Unexpectedly, my next awareness was gratitude … for the rare hoot of an owl outside my window at rhythmically-timed 30-second intervals. Even my groggy, spooning bird-dog perked up at the sound. Both of us marveled with different agendas. Nature reminded me that neither of my parents is in pain anymore. I believe they are together again. They are free. And in a way, my new status feels freeing to me as well. Still sad, but also free. More gratitude flows in. So it goes. Grieving and gratitude. Hold a space for both.

Call to Action:
Hold a space for grieving losses and gratitude each day. Even just for one minute. What will you do today?

# My Closing Thoughts

*I Send You...*

Awareness of your immeasurable value; now until you take your last breath (regardless of what you weigh or what you've eaten today).

Boundless renewed energy for daily self-care PIES.

Unshakeable faith that you are worth extreme daily self-care, even on days when you have to "fake it till you make it."

Willingness to connect with your feelings on paper.

Laughter.

The reminder that gratitude leads to acceptance (start with wacky if necessary).

Confidence to walk through fear (because amazing things are on the other side).

Connection with other women who feel the same way.

**Remember:**

- Don't waste another second being unkind to yourself or doubting yourself or playing small.

- You are being prepared to receive all the love and joy your heart can hold.

- Take the time to invest in yourself.

**Ponder:**

- Are you ready to join me and an entire community of passionate women?

- Are you ready to stop believing the lies your head tells you?

- Are you ready to start the most inspired chapter of your life?

*You're worth it!*
*You've got this!*
*We've got this!*
—SALLY

# Acknowledgments

*Life just doesn't happen by itself.* Many have offered roadmaps and support through their written words and personal support. My Role Models/Teachers/Angels include:

1. Patricia Allen, PhD, Marriage & Family Therapist

2. Louise Hay; anything by her, but especially, *Life: Reflections on Your Journey* and *Heal Your Body*

3. Ann Corwin, PhD, MEd, Family and Child Development Consultant

4. Sandy McDaniel, Family and Child Development Consultant

5. Anne Lamott, Operating Instructions

6. Ellyn Satter, any book by her, but especially *Child of Mine: Feeding With Love* and *Good Sense*

7. Elizabeth Crary, any book by her, but especially *Dealing With Disappointment: helping kids cope when things don't go their way*

8. SARK (aka Susan Ariel Rainbow Kennedy), any book by her

9. Leila Zafaranchi, MD FACOG

10. Warren Cook

11. Miranda Nguyen

12. Melissa Pearl

13. Teresa Power

14. Monica

15. Beautiful H.

16. Baxter Bartlett

# About the Author

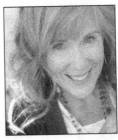

*Sally Bartlett* is an expert perimeno-pausal and menopausal coach, speaker and leader of women's online courses and retreats. She skillfully weaves together her academic and professional backgrounds with her decades-long personal experience of living in and loving the hell out of her right-sized body.

Sally earned a BA in psychology from UC Berkeley and is multi-certified by the American Council on Exercise, STOTT Pilates, and the MELT Method. For more than 20 years, she has coached women aged 16-90 to reconnect with their bodies and to reignite their passion for movement with realistic expectations and radical self-acceptance.

Her Big Amazing Life resides in Southern California.

Coming Soon:
*Dammit … It IS Menopause!*
*Companion Journal/Workbook*

# How to Work With Sally

## Online Courses:
### Level 1: The Healthy Body Mindset Recipe
Learn the Basic Ingredients for Body-Confidence in the 2nd Chapter of Your Life

Is your worth determined by your weight and your performance on your most recent diet? Do you yearn to put an end to self-loathing for the second chapter of your life, but don't know how? Develop a more current self-image with respect to aging, whether you have had body-confidence issues all your life or issues are just now arising for the first time with the onset of perimenopause. Break free from Diet Mentality.

- Identify negative self-talk that is holding you back.

- Learn a powerful journaling technique to redirect negative self-talk into positive self-talk in order to flourish.

- Find peace around food choices and freedom from dieting.

## Level 2: Finally Loving Your Body...
## How To Maintain That!

Maintaining Your Body-Confidence Through Journaling

Improve Emotional Regulation by getting current and staying current with your feelings. Learn new ways of living where you stay in touch with feelings and reignite and challenge your intellect. Are there some long-stifled passions inside just waiting to come out? Now is the time!

- Take a closer look at self-limiting beliefs and fears and negative self-talk.

- Expand on journaling strategies to develop and strengthen healthy self-talk.

- Cultivate an awareness of your actual passions that have been sabotaged by self-limiting beliefs time and time again.

Watch for exciting upcoming workshops, courses, and speeches on Sally's website: **www.SallyBartlett.com.**

# Speaking Topics

### Dammit ... It IS Menopause ... Now What?

Are you not recognizing yourself in the mirror lately?  Are you suddenly experiencing mood swings, hot flashes, forgetfulness and brain fog to name a few?

- Why Your Life is So NOT Over.

- How to make a sustained daily commitment to living in and loving a healthy-sized body for optimal quality of life and aging.

- How to take the time to invest in yourself – and why you're worth it!

### It's Never Too Late – Body-Confidence through Journaling: Imperfect Eating, Exercise & Accountability

Do you have an inner critic that just won't quit?  Learn how to use journaling techniques to acquaint yourself with a new, compassionate voice and rock your second chapter of life.

- Stop Dieting for good; learn self-compassion and find peace.

- Learn how to stop the negative shame spiral when inevitable spontaneous eating occurs.

- Right-size your mindset around exercising for the purpose of disease prevention and healthy aging, cardiovascular health, muscle strength, bone strength, balance, fighting depression, sleeping better, pain-free movement, and adding to your energy levels.

To check on Sally's availability, call, or email:
**949-285-4212**
Sally@SallyBartlett.com
www.SallyBartlett.com

## Follow Sally on:

IamSallyBartlett

@IamSallyBartlett

@ImSallyBartlett

Sally Bartlett

IamSallyBartlett

# You Might Also Enjoy

*Dammit ...*
**It IS *Menopause!***
volume 1

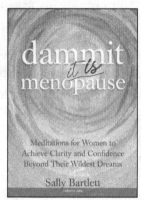

# Coming Soon

*Dammit ...* **It IS *Menopause!***
Companion Journal / Workbook

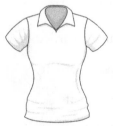

**Varsity Products:**
Varsity Transition T-shirts